OTHER FERTI[L]
SHEIL[A]

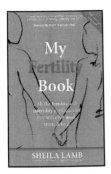

Struggling to understand the medical and non-medical fertility language? This comprehensive book explains over 200 complex terms in plain English. Available in print and ebook.

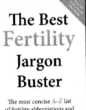

Feeling overwhelmed by the infertility language? Don't have a clue what the abbreviations and acronyms mean on fertility forums, groups and websites? All is made clear in this invaluable resource. Available in print and as a free ebook – download from www.mfsbooks.co.uk

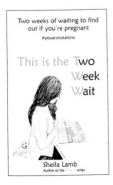

Dreading the 2WW? Don't know how you're going to get through the next 336 hours? Feel the warmth and support surround you as you read real-life experiences and thoughts from the amazing TTC community. #youarenotalone Available in print and as an ebook.

Real-life experiences from the TTC community

#youarenotalone

This is **T**rying **T**o **C**onceive

Sheila Lamb

Author of the *This is* series

Published in 2019 by MFSBooks.com

Cover Illustration Sheila Alexander

Cover Design Marketing Hand

Copy Editor Sherron Mayes, from The Editing Den

Illustrations Sheila Alexander and Phillip Reed

Print ISBN 978-1-9993035-2-5

A CIP catalogue record for this book is available from the British Library

Dedicated to all the amazing women and men in
the TTC Community

Foreword

Are you struggling to conceive and you don't know how to handle your thoughts or feelings? Do you have a family member, or partner, struggling to conceive, and you don't know what to say to them? Are you a male who doesn't have anyone to talk to about the jerk-off room?

If you answered yes to any of the above questions, then this book is the right one for you. Sheila Lamb has curated insights, advice and experiences from real people who have struggled, or are still struggling with infertility, into this amazingly helpful book, *This Is Trying to Conceive*. Composed of different entries, giving amazing points of view, and advice, on everything from how to deal with the constant barrage of unsolicited advice, to how to handle the jerk-off room, while punctuated with über-relatable illustrations and quips, this book has it all.

As the author of my own book, *Hilariously Infertile: One Woman's Inappropriate Quest to Help Other Women Through Infertility,* I am on the constant lookout for real, honest, helpful, not bogged down with medical jargon content, and *This Is Trying to Conceive* accomplishes that, and more.

The stories in this book are real and honest, not all having "happy" endings, but rather an unfiltered look into what infertility is really like. One of my favorite sections is titled, 'Seven Infertility Helpers from Hell.' This section resonated with me on such a deep level because we all know these not so helpful "helpers." From the faith based "God Reps," no explanation needed, to "The Fixer," who provides 'all' the answers, forcibly shoved down your throat, to "The Comparer," who is constantly comparing your situation to a similar situation that occurred to someone in their life that had a positive outcome. This section not only outlines these "helpers" but also sheds light on how they think, and how best to deal with, or maybe even, avoid dealing with them.

Another touching section is a poem titled, "Imagine If..."

which delves, in detail, into all the small moments that would not occur in your life if you could not have children. This section had me choking back tears on an airplane to Atlanta, Georgia; which was awkward. It was so incredibly meaningful because when I was first diagnosed with infertility, I had so many questions, and in between those questions were more personal, emotional, questions, "Would I never get pregnant? Would I never hold my own child? Would I never push my child on a swing or have a tickle fight?" This section so beautifully articulates what is going through the mind of a woman who has, for her whole life, imagined, pictured, planned, dreamed, of having a child, and then is told that she is infertile.

I commend Sheila Lamb, and all of the amazing contributors to this book, for their advice, candor, humor, and vulnerability about what life is like, 'Trying to Conceive.'

Karen Jeffries author of Hilariously Infertile

Acknowledgements

This book, and the series it is part of, would not exist, if it wasn't for the women and men who are part of the most amazing and supportive community that ever existed. It wasn't until I joined Instagram after publishing: *My Fertility Book – All the Fertility and Infertility Explanations you will ever need, from A to Z,* that I realised what 'community' actually means. Although, my rollercoaster journey ended happily several years ago, it has helped me to accept the emotions that come with infertility, and are still part of me.

My thanks, firstly, go to my miracle, rainbow daughter Jessica, who means the world to me and is my reason for writing and helping the TTC community. This book wouldn't exist if it weren't for the following people who have contributed. Some I have known for many years and met at various fertility events, and others I have only 'met' through the Instagram community. So, in alphabetical order: Alice Rose, Amber Woodward, Amelia Freeman, Amira Posner, Anon Freedom Fertility Coach, Becky Kearns, Claire Caldow, Dany Griffiths, Dr Deborah Simmons, @eggainst_the_odds, Eleanor Modral-Gibbons, @fertility_help-hub, Gareth James, Helena Tubridy, @Herfertilitydiary, Justine Bold, Karmann Wennerlind, Kate Davies, Lauren Manaker, Lianne Baker, Nicola Salmon, Rachel Cathan, Salise Wright, Sandi Friedlos, Sarah Rollandini, Stephanie Roth, @the. swim.team, Tori Day and Vince.

The book cover was illustrated by the author and illustrator, Sheila Alexander, who was so supportive and patient as I stumbled to explain what I wanted for this book and the series. We both, very much hope, you relate to the couple and their furbaby on their TTC journey.

Sheila Alexander is the author of: *IF: A Memoir of Infertility*, a graphic novel about her infertility treatment using in-vitro fertilization (IVF). She lives in Massachusetts with her husband, son, dog, and parrot. She holds a master's degree in education and is a minor in fine art from Lesley University. By day, she works as a teacher, where she shares her love of comic books with her students. She believes that books have the power to change lives, so she published her first book, in the hope that it will help other people going through infertility treatments. For more information visit her website: www.sheilaalexanderart.com or follow her on Instagram, @sheilaalexanderart.

Sheila also captured parts of this journey in the illustrations you'll find inside the book, as did the illustrator Phillip Reed, who created the illustrations in *My Fertility Book* and *This Is The Two Week Wait*. He can be contacted on info@phillipreed.net or follow on Instagram @phillipreed

I'd also like to thank the following who have encouraged and supported me to put my 'This Is' series of books together: Paul Lamb, Michelle Starkey, Claudia Sievers, Angie Conlon, Maria Bagao, Judy Marell, Lisa Bond, Jessica Hepburn, Anya Sizer, Cat Strawbridge, Emma Brodzinski, Angela Heap, Diane Chandler, @mrskmeaks, @mrandmrsivf, and @hopemattersalways.

Contents

Introduction

If you find yourself reading this book, you have my heartfelt support, because potentially you've been trying to become pregnant and have a baby for quite some time. Or, perhaps you're reading it because someone you care about has gifted it to you, or maybe it was recommended to you, so that you can understand what it's really like to cope with infertility.

The World Health Organisation says the following: "Infertility is defined as 'a disease of the reproductive system' and results in disability". Secondary infertility, which is when a woman has had at least one live baby, is more common than primary infertility, which is when a woman hasn't had a biological baby. Infertility affects roughly one in seven couples worldwide, and like all diseases, a person 'lives' with it all day, every day. Myself, and all the people who have had a 'trying to conceive' journey, really hope that this book helps you to appreciate what our life is like, so that you will be in a much better position to offer support, how and when it's needed.

I was one of those 'one in seven' and our 'trying to conceive' journey lasted about six years. When you get past four or five years, it all becomes a bit of a blur, and a week and a month all merge together, and, before you know it, another year has passed.

Anyway, I was forty years young and my husband twenty-nine when we started 'trying' for a baby, and like most couples, we thought it would happen in the first month of trying. Why shouldn't it? It didn't! Then, we thought, okay, it'll happen in the next month, won't it? It didn't! I lost count of the number of times I had that conversation in my head.

So, our fertility CV/resume reads like this:

After a year of trying to conceive, I received a diagnosis of unexplained infertility.

I had an intrauterine insemination (IUI) that was unsuccessful.

I underwent an intracytoplasmic sperm injection cycle (ISCSI) with pre-implantation screening (PGS), that was also unsuccessful.

I spent a couple of years trying to conceive naturally with Traditional Chinese medicine, acupuncture, no alcohol, took supplements, underwent hypnotherapy and reflexology – all unsuccessful.

I had a donor egg ICSI cycle that was briefly successful, but I had an early miscarriage.

I had investigations into natural killer cells and thrombophilia that all came back negative.

I underwent a donor egg ICSI cycle with aspirin, steroid and Clexane.

And then, finally … when we thought the odds were stacked against us, our beautiful rainbow daughter arrived.

Not everyone, who struggles to have a baby, goes down the route of fertility treatments like in-vitro fertilisation or IVF. But, bear in mind, that even if a couple have undergone IVF, for example – if the treatment hasn't been successful, before they decide to do another treatment, they are still coping with infertility; it doesn't just disappear, which is why some contributions touch on fertility treatment.

Many couples will conceive naturally, eventually. In 2017, it was estimated that fifty million couples worldwide experienced infertility. The NHS stats reveal that 92% of women – aged between 19 to 26 – will conceive after one year of trying, and 98% after two years. 82% of women – aged 35 to 39 – will conceive after one year of trying, and 90% after two years. It's likely that this is a comparable percentage in all developed countries. But when you're trying to conceive and it doesn't happen straight away or within the first couple of months, the worry and anxiety sets in quickly.

Finding it challenging to have a baby is a life changing experience for most. It certainly was for me. Even though we were eventually successful, this experience was very much part of my life and what made me, me. Like a lot of people who have a life changing experience, I wanted to give something back to those who also found themselves on this path, to offer help and support. So, I started an online magazine called: *My Fertility Specialist* – and the fertility experts who wrote articles, along with the women who shared their real-life stories were inspirational.

We put together eight issues over two years, and in that time, I started a spreadsheet of all the topics we could utilise for articles and listed them from A to Z. Then I realised that maybe all this information would be better in a book; a jargon-free glossary of all the medical and non-medical terms that people, without a medical degree, could understand in order to steer their journey in the direction they wanted it to take. I put the magazine on hold and concentrated on writing: *My Fertility Book: all the fertility and infertility explanations you will ever need, from A to Z* and published it in November 2019.

Most fertility terms have acronyms or are abbreviated, such as AMH, BBT, and 6DP5DT, and are often used on social media, forums, online groups and websites, so I wrote a free eBook called: *The Best Fertility Jargon Buster: the most concise A-Z list of fertility abbreviations and acronyms you will ever need.* More information can be found at the back of this book.

When we were desperately trying to conceive, even before doing fertility treatments, the emotional aspect of coping with the highs and lows was rarely discussed. On the forum that I occasionally logged into, most posts were asking for advice about tests, investigations, results and fertility treatments. I was very open with family, friends and sometimes strangers, about our struggle and was lucky, if that's the right word, to have a couple of friends who were also trying to get pregnant, so I was able to talk about my feelings with someone other than my husband. This has now changed to a certain degree, in that both women and men, along with celebrities, are more open about sharing the emotional side of infertility – the fear that they'll never become pregnant, or the distress when hearing that a friend has announced that they're pregnant, and how they're having a crap day because their period arrived.

However, there are still many people who don't feel they can share with their nearest and dearest, because they don't want people to feel sorry for them, or worry, but also, because they know they might not understand. That's why many people find support and comfort online with strangers who potentially become friends. Sharing feelings is comforting as you realise that you're not alone, and that it's okay to feel sad, angry, frustrated, impatient, jealous, and depressed. I could see on social media that women and men felt supported, boosted and, most important, felt understood and validated by a community of other people who also found themselves part of this intimate global group. Nobody wants to be in a group of seeming 'failure to conceive' people, but when you find yourself part of it, boy, are you taken care of!

It was this that gave me the idea of putting all these lovely, warm, supportive, virtual hugging words into a book. Then if you wake at 3 a.m., and can't get back to sleep, because all you can think is 'why aren't I pregnant yet?' reach for this book and read what other like-minded people have to say.

Practically all the contributors have had their own infertility challenges, and if they haven't, they have worked with people who have been trying to conceive for many years. They've kindly given up their time to share their own experience of infertility for this book. Each quoted extract is in the voice of the contributor.

Remember, there is no right or wrong way to deal with this journey, but these inspiring women and men all wanted to share some nuggets of inspiration, hopes, fears and their joy, in the hope that what they'll say will in some way help – until you hold your longed-for baby in your arms, and start your lives together as a family.

A letter to someone who's trying to conceive

Dear Friend,

Come here and let me give you a big virtual hug. Trying to Conceive (TTC) can be demoralising and painful at times. It does things to your mind – makes you feel ashamed, unworthy, anxious, and depressed – and no one, ever, should have to go through it. Sadly, though, you're not alone as you'll read in this book.

Most of the contributors, men and women, have had, or are still experiencing rollercoaster fertility challenges themselves. They have written from their heart, about what was, or still is, important to them about their journey. I contacted each contributor and told them I was writing a series of books to support the TTC community, and would they like to contribute by sharing their experience – the good, the bad and the ugly – and because they know how important having support is, and that we are all much stronger together, they said 'Yes!'

Although, I expect, it will be mostly women who read this book, there are contributions from men, so please share with your man. If you haven't told your family and friends about TTC yet, because you don't know how to start the conversation, maybe it would help if you gave them a copy of this book and just tiptoe away, leaving them to read while you make a cup of tea/coffee. Or if you've told family and friends, and they are consistently unsupportive, saying insensitive things, such as that old chestnut: 'just relax, it will happen', perhaps give them a copy with some highlighted contributions that you think will help them empathise. You could start with the letter that has been written to the 'Don't get it brigade' on the next page and the excerpts from Alice's 'Think! What Not To Say' campaign videos; #humourandcompassion.

Although our experiences might be different, our emotions can be pretty similar: sadness, anxiety, anger, jealousy, and, oh, the frustrating impatience of endlessly waiting for results. If you're at the beginning of your journey, you may wonder if it's only you who feels jealous of your BFFs pregnancy announcement, or how your life seems to revolve around ovulation, sex, and menstrual periods. 'Where has the fun and laughter gone?' you might ask. It's important that you acknowledge these feelings, and not let them overwhelm you.

There are a number of ways of finding the support that is right for you, and with every contribution is the person's Instagram name, and they'll be very happy to welcome you to the TTC community. If the contribution is by someone who helps the community professionally, at the back of the book is a 'Resources' section, if you want to connect with them.

The most important thing to remember is that you're not alone on your journey.

Lots of love,

Sheila and the TTC community

A letter to someone who hasn't experienced infertility

Dear Friend,

Firstly, thank you so much for opening this book. It's probably not the sort of book you'd normally read, but, please, read some of it. I hope you don't mind me starting with the boring, but essential part first. Most people are shocked and surprised when they find out that one in eight couples find it challenging to have a baby, and that the World Health Organisation (WHO) recognises infertility as a disease. In one third of infertile couples, infertility is a complication with the man; in one third, it's a complication with the woman, and in one third, it's with both – or the problem can't be identified. Couples in their twenties, thirties and forties can all face the challenge of infertility. If you know six or seven couples, there's a big likelihood that one of them is dealing with infertility, but you won't necessarily be aware of this unless they tell you.

For a number of reasons, many keep infertility to themselves often through embarrassment, shame, or that they simply don't want to worry you. It's a deeply personal thing, and to be honest, they keep hoping that they'll fall pregnant the following month, then they won't ever have to tell you.

It's not easy to talk about something like this, so if someone has given you this book to read, it's because they want you to know what they are going through. They'll hope that you'll understand their emotions and not judge them. They won't want your sympathy or pity, they'll just want their feelings validated, and for you to understand better, so you can perhaps offer some support. Don't be that friend or family member who turns away from someone who needs a hug, or worse, says something insensitive.

Throughout the book you'll read excerpts taken from Alice Rose's 'Think! What Not To Say' campaign videos, which aim to educate the wider world about how to support someone going through a fertility journey. By opening a dialogue – with humour and compassion (which Alice has in abundance) – between patient, practitioners, family, friends, colleagues and anyone in patient facing roles, we can start to break down stigmas, normalise fertility conversations across the board, and start to encourage better communication from all sides. The more we talk about it, the easier it will be for all of us.

So, how does a person who's dealing with infertility cope on a daily basis? No, wait, sometimes on an hourly basis. Well, they can wake up one morning feeling happy and positive, then they see another pregnancy announcement or get invited to a baby shower, and suddenly they are overcome with sadness for themselves, their partner, their family and friends, because, it isn't them announcing their pregnancy and sending invites to their baby shower. You may think they're being selfish, or they shouldn't be jealous, and you're right – but they can't help it. Have you ever been jealous of someone even if you loved them? Maybe, they got a fantastic job they wanted, whilst you were still in the job, you disliked. Maybe they just got married, and you were about to get separated or divorced. Not quite the same thing, I know, but you get my drift about jealousy.

You will read about people who have gone through, or are still going through infertility, or 'trying to conceive (TTC)' as we say in our community. Their experiences will help others who are TTC, but what we all really want is for people who haven't struggled to have a baby, to really understand and maybe 'get it'. Although we are all on different journeys to have our much-wanted babies, how we feel is often very much the same. We are a community and we support each other completely. And we hope you get to meet our baby that we have fought so hard for, very, very soon.

Lots of love,

Sheila and The TTC Community

Offer the support you would want if it were you

There is nothing in the world quite like the challenge of having a baby. I say 'having a baby' because all too often a pregnancy ends in a miscarriage whether it's the first month or the twenty fourth month of trying. So, I never say I'm 'getting pregnant' because the dream is to have a baby. Why do I say there's nothing else in the world – because making a baby takes two people in some shape or form. Most other diseases (and yes, the WHO recognise infertility as a disease), that I'm aware of directly only affect the one person who has the actual disease. I agree that of course their family and friends are affected by the person having the disease, but the family and friends probably don't blame themselves, or actually live with it emotionally every day, like the person who has the disease does.

Studies show that the stress and anxiety of infertility is the same as someone who has cancer. Yes, they are two very different things, but no one would imagine for a minute that cancer doesn't cause stress and anxiety, yet people are often surprised to hear the same when someone talks about their infertility. The stress of infertility comes from the uncertainty and emotional upheaval experienced by the couple in their day-to-day world.

I've tried to think of an analogy that may explain infertility better than I can using just words. Let's give it a go. At some point in your life you were single. It may have been years ago, but try to remember back to those days. Maybe, when you were single, everyone else you knew was in a relationship, and they then went on to get engaged and married. Remember how you felt? Did you feel sad, depressed, angry, upset, and jealous, and think you'd never find someone? Did you go on dates, maybe, a lot of dates? You were excited at the thought of going on the date, planning what you'd wear, constantly thinking about how the date would go. Sound familiar? But the date didn't work out; you don't know why exactly, but it didn't, and you felt down and sad after, as you thought 'this was the one'. But you picked yourself up and dated again in the hope that this date would be 'the one'. Imagine this happening every month when you're trying to get pregnant – the build-up during the month of having sex regularly, but especially around the time you ovulate – no pressure! Then the waiting for ten days to two weeks to find out if this month you're pregnant. But your period arrives and you're not pregnant. You don't know why, because this is what everyone else does and they get pregnant. The dating analogy is sort of what it's like – but multiply the feelings and emotions by 100% and you're getting close.

Sticking with the being single analogy, while all your friends are dating, getting engaged and married, did you ever feel sorry for yourself, complain that you can't find 'the one'? Not all the time, of course, but you're only human and it's natural to prefer to be in a relationship than to be single – though there's always an exception to the rule. Did you mind that your great aunt Agnes said to you "You're trying too hard. Stop looking and you'll meet someone," – and you're thinking, 'doesn't she realise it's different nowadays to back in her day?' – or your annoying cousin who's always dating a different person every month said: "Go on Cantfindtheone.com, there's plenty of single people on there. That's where I always find my next girl/boyfriend," (grrrrrrr, I don't want your cast-offs!). Did you plaster a smile on your face when secretly all you wanted to do was stick your tongue out at great aunt Agnes and smack the smug cousin in the face? It hurts when people don't acknowledge your feelings. They brush them away as if they don't matter and aren't important, and you don't feel supported in any shape or form.

Exactly the same thing happens to people when they're trying to get pregnant. They hear things like "You're trying too hard; don't think about it; go on holiday; get a dog or cat, then it'll happen." And you might think '"will it, even though I have a low sperm count?", or "Have you heard about <insert latest super food here>, my work colleague's, next door neighbour's, best friend's sister's cousin ate this and she got pregnant in a month." And the answer might be: "that's interesting, the last I heard, said 'super food' can't do anything for endometriosis!" But the worse one is "You can have one of mine!" And you're thinking, "Why would I want your child? Just like you, we want a child of our own".

So just like a single person looking for the love of their life, there are no guarantees they will find them. There are no guarantees that someone will ever have the baby they long for. But while they are trying, whether it's for three years, or six or fifteen, please, realise how brave that woman and man are to put themselves through such an emotional, draining, exhausting time in order to have their baby. You should be very proud of them, and support them exactly how you would like to be supported if it were you.

Sheila @fertilitybooks

Telling others about infertility

The people you expect to be able to talk to about infertility, sadly, aren't always the ones that will listen.

I've often felt the need to talk about it in an optimistic light to close friends and family despite feeling extremely pessimistic. It's as if I have a responsibility not to make them feel bad or awkward by letting them know that I'm struggling, or that it won't work out. Strangely, perhaps, I've found it easier to talk about it with people I don't know as well, because they're less invested in me and my partner's fertility journey.

I have a really strong memory of chatting to a guy I once played football with about our attempts to get pregnant – we were probably three or so years into our fertility journey. We talked for a good while about it really openly, and despite nothing being different at the end of our chat, I felt much better about things, having been able to share how I was feeling. A couple of weeks later he told me that his wife was pregnant, and he felt really bad, as they hadn't been trying and it wasn't in their immediate plans. But I didn't feel remotely negative about their news, as the opportunity I'd had to discuss it with him, felt like something which had been really important to us both. I think it opened his eyes to how fertility isn't a given, but also gave me a chance to talk openly and air some things I hadn't really talked about with anyone, not even my wife.

The key to discussing fertility is for the other person to have a willingness to listen and an awareness that they can't solve the problem. When discussing our fertility issues with friends and family, I never wanted their advice on what decision we should make next, or assertions that we'd be successful in time. I just wanted them to allow me to explain what was happening and how that was making me feel. Men often don't have many opportunities to express their feelings, so being given an opportunity to do that is really important. That's not solely in relation to fertility either. Going through this has made me more conscious of checking in with my friends and genuinely asking them how they're doing, rather than the standard social pleasantries. It's not always an easy thing to do, but if you approach it with genuine interest and a willingness to listen, you can't go far wrong.

Vince

From the 'Think! What Not To Say' campaign videos

"Just RELAX"

Of course, relaxing would be beneficial, just as every single person in the world probably needs to relax a bit with whatever they're going through. But this is probably the top culprit! It's like telling an angry person to calm down. PLEASE, PLEASE don't say this!

#humourandcompassion

Alice Rose @thisisalicerose

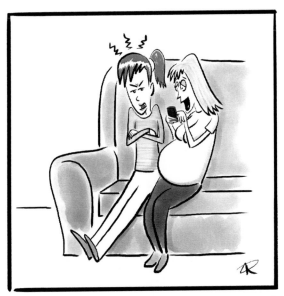

"Try this app, I used it and got pregnant within a month of downloading it!"

Life before infertility

Do you remember your life, before infertility? Do you remember what you loved to do, your passions, your drive? Do you remember the joy you had when it was just the two of you? What did you love to do together?

Infertility can start to become our only focus. We start to forget who we are as an individual and as a couple. Some of us try for a family right away, only to find ourselves being sucked into a dark abyss. Some take time as a couple before trying, not knowing it will be a long haul. No matter how you go about it, infertility consumes us in every way.

We started trying early on in our marriage, and it took me away from who I really was. Ryan was better at keeping his priorities, but it wasn't easy. The one thing I am so grateful for was our time together and getting away. After each loss or setback, we took vacations, and it gave me something to look forward to.

The WAITING is what drags you down and pushes the feelings of depression and anxiety to an all-time high. I found that when I had something exciting to count down to, it helped ease the pain and sorrow. It's what 'saved me' over those ten years of waiting to become a mom.

Ryan pushed me to go back to school and get my Master's in Early Childhood Special Education. I was thankful he helped me to not lose myself completely.

We loved trying new restaurants and eating yummy food. It became our goal to not eat at the same place and be as adventurous as possible. It's created some of my greatest memories. We tried to do things that brought joy together amongst the heartache. It helped us remember what it was like before the stress took over.
What are the things you love to do?
What things do you do together to find joy?

Karmenn Wennerlind @karmennwennerlind

Be kind

Struggling with infertility over the years has taught me many important lessons — how to listen to my body; how to be patient as meaningful change happens gradually over time; how important it is to tackle stress as daily struggles are so unimportant that they will be forgotten the following week; how to change my expectations, as nothing happens as and when you hope it will. But above all, infertility has taught me to be kind, because you never know the secret struggles of others.

People probably looked at me throughout my 'dark years' of infertility and thought that I had got it together, happily winning at life like the smug thirty-something career driven urbanite that we all know and love. But I was a mess. I could barely get out of bed. I cried every week and became a hermit – a total and utter shambles. I refused to disclose this aspect of myself outside of my inner circle, which consisted of my husband and our cat. So now, whenever I see someone who seemingly has it all, I gently remind myself to be kind, as I have no idea of their secret struggles. And everyone has something, some private fight that nobody sees. And so, I always tell myself, 'BE KIND'.

Amber Woodward @thepreggerskitchen

Imagine if....

You'd never seen two lines on a pregnancy test stick.

You'd never be able to say to your partner "I'm pregnant!"

You'd never heard or seen your baby's heartbeat on the ultrasound scan.

You'd never seen your baby playing hide-n-seek or waving at you on your ultrasound scan.

You'd never been able to tell family and friends that you're pregnant/expecting a baby.

You'd never felt your baby move inside your womb.

You'd never been able to place your partner's hand on your belly so they could feel your baby move.

You'd never been asked if you want to know the sex of your baby.

You'd never been able to attend your own baby shower.

You'd never get to give your baby the name you and your partner had chosen.

You'd never gone to the shop to choose a pram and practiced pushing it around the shop with a grin from ear to ear.

You'd never chosen colours, nursery furniture and accessories for your baby's nursery.

You'd never heard the midwife or doctor say "It's a girl!" or "It's a boy!"

You'd never heard your baby's first cry.

You'd never given your baby their first cuddle.

You'd never given your baby a kiss goodnight.

You'd never felt your baby's soft, downy, warm skin against your skin.

You'd never seen your baby's first smile.

You'd never told everyone your baby has his or her first tooth.

You'd never heard your baby say "Mamma" or "Dadda."

You'd never received your first Mother's Day or Father's Day card.

You'd never experienced your baby holding out their arms for a cuddle from you.

You'd never played peek-a-boo with your child and seen the happiness on their face.

You'd never seen your baby crawl for the first time.

You'd never taken your baby to the shoe shop for their first pair of shoes.

You'd never seen your baby cruise, walk or run for the first time.

You'd never heard your child say "I love you, Mummy" or "I

love you, Daddy."

You'd never comforted your child when they're sad.

You'd never cried at your child's first day at nursery or school.

You'd never held your child's hand as you walk down the street together.

You'd never jumped in muddy puddles with your child.

You'd never placed their first tooth under their pillow for the tooth fairy.

Imagine, if you didn't have all your memories of these precious moments with your child or children.

Imagine what it's like for me, so desperate to experience all that you have, but not knowing if I'll ever have these memories.

Sheila @fertilitybooks

From the 'Think! What Not To Say' campaign videos

"My friend went on holiday and stopped trying … and it happened! Have you thought about booking a holiday?"

Even if you do hear of this happening, and even if there's something in it, it is, again, completely infuriating - it implies the person is failing at 'trying' to get pregnant as well as actually failing to 'get' pregnant because they haven't been on holiday yet!"

#humourandcompassion

Alice Rose @thisisalicerose

Finding support

I'm in a male only Facebook group which does help with offering support. However, my wife and I would love to meet couples in the same situation, but we can't find any. We have friends who've been through fertility treatment, but most were successful first time. We are the only couple who are still childless. It's difficult to talk to couples who have children as there is no way they can relate to the pain of not having a child. Our female friends have been very supportive and I can talk to women far easier than men. For some reason, it's harder for me to share with men. Only my really close male friends know what we've been through and they always ask, but they both have kids, (again not their fault), but I'd share more and find it more helpful to talk to couples in the same position as us. We are both very open about our struggles and would attend face to face support, but we don't know where that's available.

Gareth James, UK

Secondary infertiltity sucks too

Secondary infertility — where the woman has given birth to at least one live baby — is as common as primary infertility — where the woman hasn't given birth to a biological baby. It's estimated that one in six couples who already have at least one child, fail to get pregnant within one year of having unprotected sex.

Couples experiencing secondary infertility have the same feelings about their infertility as couples who are trying to have their first baby. Their feelings run along the same lines, and people often don't realise this.

Jealousy – of the women who plan their subsequent pregnancies and get pregnant when they want.

Guilty – for feeling insanely jealous of the above (how is it even possible to feel both these emotions at the same time!)

Frustration – that their body has done it before, why can't it do it again?

Sadness – at not being able to give their child/children what they innocently ask for: a baby brother/sister.

They also face the same insensitive comments from those who don't 'get it', such as 'just relax', 'go on holiday', 'lose some weight'. However, they also hear 'at least you have one child', 'you have so much to be thankful for, some people struggle to have just one'.

They know they have so much to be thankful for, they don't need telling, thank you, and they do feel horribly guilty for having these feelings, especially when they might know people who haven't been able to have a child. And like these people, they are grieving the family and life they had planned and dreamed of, and they deserve their feelings and grief to be validated. (See: 'The Grief of Infertility'). People with secondary infertility are just as likely to keep this private from family and friends because of these comments and the lack of understanding.

What's different for those going through secondary infertility is that they feel they are in no-man's land. Often their friends and other mums they know at the school gates are discussing the ideal age gap between children. Do they comment or not, because they aren't having any choice over this at the moment? It's been taken out of their control, and like infertility, it sucks big time. Another indecision is: do they get rid of the baby gear and clothes that they've had hanging around, because they just don't know if they will ever use them again.

There are face to face support groups and online groups specifically for those going through secondary infertility, because the emotions are different to primary infertility. Also, a lot of times, women with secondary infertility can feel awkward talking about their infertility to someone who is struggling to have their first baby, although they have no need to feel like this. Infertility is infertility; however, you look at it.

Sheila @fertilitybooks

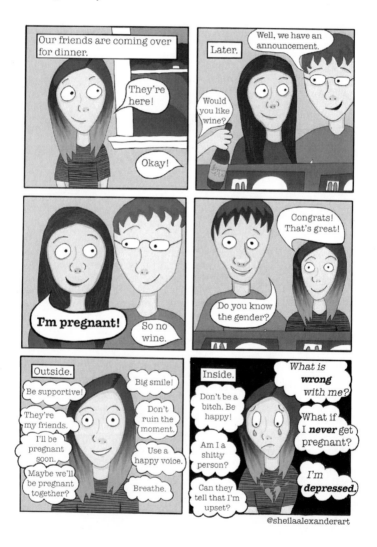

@sheilaalexanderart

34

From the blog: 'Seven Infertility Helpers from Hell'

If you are going through infertility, I am absolutely certain that you've come across at least one, if not more, infertility helpers from hell. If you know someone whose going through infertility, then you may, or may not, recognise yourself as an infertility helper from hell. Sorry, I don't mean to offend you. An infertility helper from hell is a person who means well, but who hinders your healing. Their intentions may be good, but their efforts often turn out to be self-absorbed and, ultimately, unhelpful. Here I respectfully offer, 'Seven Infertility Helpers from Hell'.

1. **The Fixer**—The Fixer is certain that your terrible situation is a question and they know the answer. In fact, this person has ALL the answers to how to heal from your predicament. Note that I called this a predicament, not your fear and pain. For them, this is a project to be figured out. There's a blueprint. Just do what they recommend, be grateful, and you will be A-OK. Doesn't that make you feel all warm and fuzzy from your head to your toes? And you better feel good real quick. I remember when The Fixer told my husband and me to make love on the beach under a full moon and we'd get pregnant. I couldn't make this up. The answer has been offered. What are you waiting for? Get to it. And Don't-Worry-About-It! Unfortunately, your spouse may be a Fixer. The Fixer needs you to take their advice and feel good, because he or she is already thinking about their own life, and it's too difficult to even imagine what you're going through. They can't. They'd rather work on you as a goodwill project than consider the possibility of fear and pain in their own lives.

2. **The Comparer**—The Comparer knows a person with PCOS who GOT PREGNANT on their FIRST IVF cycle and then they GOT PREGNANT again ON THEIR OWN and they KNOW that you will too! They don't know how they know this, but they sure do. Because the Comparer refuses to accept that your predicament is personal—and yes, (ahem) many vaginal ultrasounds and semen samples are personal — this person needs to deflect your personal pain. It would be really painful for this person to feel your pain. This person will not win a gold medal in validation or empathy. They file you into a category for which they have a reference. They may also talk about how they are the same as you, because something really bad happened to them in their life, like whiplash, or they didn't get that job they really wanted. And they were very, very sad. FYI, your pain is about them, too. The Comparer can't deal with the intense feelings that you are dealing with, and it's easier to talk about themselves or someone else who also has a really, really, really hard story. Even harder than your own, of course.

3. **The Reporter**—The Reporter wants all the juicy details. "Oooooh, tell me more?" they say. They have many questions, ranging from the curious to the spicy, and they await your detailed answers. This is a Pulitzer prize winning *New York Times* reporter with a spiral notebook and a digital recorder. And once The Reporter has the data, they just CANNOT keep a secret. They have to share your big, horrible story with others without your consent. "Did you hear? Isn't that JUST AWFUL?" The Reporter shares with boundaryless abandon in the spirit of transparency, because she or he is just so darn worried about you. Really, it's easier to tell a story than to feel your pain.

4. **The Cricket**—*sound of crickets*. I am whispering. This person is quiet because they don't know what to do, or say, or ask. They don't want to do anything that might make you feel worse. So, they do nothing. But they may say they heard you were doing okay, from The Reporter maybe? And they are hoping against hope that that's true, because they don't know what to do, or say, or ask.

5. **God Reps**—Everybody take a breath and please don't curse me out. I'm just a messenger here. The God Rep is on a gossamer trail of thoughts and prayers, straight from The Big One upstairs. This person knows how you should feel. Isn't that a relief? God knows why you are in this predicament, according to the God Rep. They feel called upon by the Lord to tell you that God has a plan for you. The suffering of trying to conceive for years and spending a bucket of money on having children is part of the plan. Isn't it that simple? I have seen many good people, devout people, get violently furious about the God Rep's very important message. Did you know that you can have a conversation with God directly, without the God Rep's 'help', and that you can feel, however you feel, good or bad? The Big One can handle all of your feelings.

6. **The Cheerleader**—Yay! You are going to be okay! They just know it! Turn that frown upside down! Rah! You have time! You are young! You are going to beat the odds! This is gonna work! You just gotta think positive! You just need to put on your lipstick and 'relax and eat your vegetables and do acupuncture!' The Cheerleader is too uncomfortable to step out of their rosy formation to consider your reality. They don't understand that they are dismissing your every emotion and leaving you feeling quite alone.

7. **The Victim**—The Victim has heard about your terrible news and feels just awful — wait for it — that you didn't share your news directly with them. They had to hear second-hand. They are overcome with emotion. They are so distraught about being left out of your big story that they need to breathe for a moment. They thought you were close. They need to tell you how they feel. Please note that they haven't expressed any empathy for YOUR frustration and grief. Theirs is bigger. Much bigger.

Who is the Real Helper when you feel vulnerable and afraid?

It's the person who just listens, who gives you a hug without offering advice. The Real Helper goes to the clinic with you, just because. They cry with you, because infertility is unfair, and they know you hurt. It's the person who offers understanding, not judgment. They ask and understand when you can't talk about it today. They hold out hope for you, and your future when you feel hopeless. They don't offer to give you one of their children. They give what they can give in the hope that it's helpful to you somehow, maybe now, maybe later. And this person keeps checking in, offering a smile or an open ear.

Sometimes you have to be very clear with people about what you need. Like me, East Coast Debbie. In the words of the immortal Spice Girls, "I'll tell you what I want, what I really, really want." What most people are desperate for is EMPATHY. The Real Helpers do exist. Please take the risk and open your heart to them.

Dr Deborah Simmons @partners_in_fertility

The grief of infertility

The pain of infertility is often unrecognised by those who haven't gone through their own journey, and therefore, the grief for the children you hold in your heart is quite unique. Others, don't get it, because there is nothing tangible or real to grieve – as far as they can see, what you're grieving for hasn't actually happened yet. But it's real, because you've lived with your dreams for a family, you decided how you'll make your pregnancy announcement, decided on your children's names, decided how you'll decorate the nursery and much more – and when it hasn't happened yet, you are in pain and grieving.

Did you know that there are scholarly terms to describe this type of grief?

- Disenfranchised Grief – losses that others don't acknowledge, so think you don't have the right to grieve. Is there a Hallmark card for it? No, then it's a disenfranchised loss.
- Ambiguous Grief – losses in which others are not sure you've had a loss, but you believe you've had a loss.

This lack of other people not recognising our loss, makes it easy for us to feel that we aren't entitled to grieve. If you've told others about your infertility journey, then some of the comments you receive can be the kind that make you want to stab the person in the eye with a red-hot poker. Any of the following sound familiar? 'Kids aren't all they're cracked up to be', 'you can always adopt' 'you get to enjoy adult holidays/a tidy house/go to the loo without being interrupted' or 'be grateful you have your health'. What these people are basically saying to you is buck up and get over it. Thanks for nothing.

This is very unfair because grief and loss cannot and should not be compared. Yes, you are lucky to have a tidy house, but just because you do, doesn't mean you can't feel sad that you don't have the little people to make your house messy.

As well as grieving a dream, you are also grieving a marker for conversation. How often have you met someone new who quickly asks if you have children, because this is what people ask to get a conversation going? Either they ask about children or what do you do for a job? So, you are also grieving the ability to have conversations with people about children, because you don't have them.

Having the support of others in recognising our loss, enables us to address our loss, and share our loss that we don't have children yet. Validating our loss can be very important for many and it makes it easier for us to live with this loss. There are usually triggering events that bring grief to the surface, such as pregnancy announcements, an invite to a baby shower, holiday times where there'll be babies and children. To help with the grief, acknowledge to yourself that the situation is likely to cause you grief by understanding why does this event hurt, why do people ask questions as to when you are going to have children; often they are just making conversation or are curious. And think about how you might answer their question – you may be polite or not so polite, i.e. snarky, or just deflect it, it's totally up to you. If you can't bring yourself to be snarky to their face, you can certainly say snarky retorts in your head – doesn't this help to control your anger!

The most important thing in getting through loss and grief and coming out intact the other side, is having hope and support. Research has shown that people who are grieving any sort of loss and are able to identify some aspect of hopefulness, move through grief with a better outcome. It may be that right now feeling hopeful is hard; even being hopeful that you get out of bed today is enough, or you hope that tomorrow is better than today. Finding non-judgemental support – wherever that may be – will enable you to express and explore your feelings, because they are as justified as the next persons.

Sheila @fertilitybooks

From worrier to warrior

When navigating a fertility journey there is so much to think about, consider and quite frankly – worry about!

It doesn't have to be that way though. I teach my IVF coaching clients to adapt an 80/20 rule. 80% of their time they endeavour to live their life, and 20% of their time is for thinking, researching and worrying about fertility. However, to do this you need to train your brain to worry when you want to, and not allow worrying to be the boss of you. My coaching tool 'From Worrier to Warrior' is a firm favourite with my clients. This tool not only takes charge of your worries, but it helps you take action to deal with your worries and embrace the 80/20 rule.

1. **Build a habit of deliberate worry**

   Choose a place that you intend to spend your time worrying in each day. This could be a worry chair or a particular room (never the bedroom). Come to this place at a set time each day to worry/research/think. By doing so, you are training your mind to understand that YOU are in charge and your worries are not the boss of you. You're not suppressing your worries, simply postponing them until you are ready to deal with them.

2. Create a worry list

In your worry place, get onto paper all the things that are troubling you, but also write down any research you may need to do, or actions you might need to take. Take a few minutes to free write and don't judge your thoughts. Crazy is good!

3. Categorise your worries

Use a traffic light system to organise your worries:

Green Worries – worries that need to be solved and are immediate and pressing. There's evidence that what you are worried about is true.

To overcome 'Green Worries' you need to ACT. Make a decision on what you need to do, set a deadline and do it! Don't procrastinate, as action needs to be taken to remove this worry.

Amber Worries – worries that are imaginary, the 'what if's'. It's likely that you'll have a lot of these. These are worries about a future event that you may or may not be able to control.

To overcome 'Amber Worries' you need to plan. Start devising an action plan to ease this worry. You can include things that you need to research or questions you need to ask. Stick to your plan to move forward with this worry.

Red Worries – worries that you cannot control or answer. Red Worries include worrying about what someone else might think, feel, say or do.

To overcome 'Red Worries' embrace uncertainty and know that you are not responsible for other people and cannot control their actions or thoughts.

Learning to take back control of your worries takes time. The more you can practice, the easier and more natural it will become. Remember, fertility is part of you, but by no means all of you. And, now, is the time to start living your life.

Kate Davies @your_fertility_journey

Breaking the taboo of infertility

Talking about TTC isn't something that comes naturally to most – it seems that there is an unwritten rule that it's never to be spoken of, whether it be a natural conception or an assisted conception. Because of this, it's become a vicious cycle – *nobody talks about infertility*, and so we worry about people's reactions, and because we think that people will react negatively, we don't say anything, therefore perpetuating the cycle. This really doesn't help the feeling of isolation, that you're alone in your struggle to conceive, and are unable to share this with your friends and family for fear of a lack of understanding and unwanted reactions.

I tell my story openly to try and break this taboo for future parents-to-be who are struggling to conceive. I want to raise awareness that it's actually quite common to conceive with a little help from science – in fact one in six couples in the UK have trouble conceiving – and to show people that it's nothing to be ashamed of or embarrassed about. Since 'coming out' of the infertility closet I can honestly say that I haven't received any negative reactions. By far, the majority have been overwhelmingly positive and supportive. From time to time, however, some reactions have unknowingly revealed the remaining underlying taboos and embarrassment that still surround the topic of assisted conception.

As an example, I took one of my three donor conceived IVF daughters, Eska, to the Out of Hours GP at our local hospital. The gentleman on reception commented on how lovely and unusual her name was, followed by a totally innocent question about its origin. I replied happily, as I always do, by telling him that we had IVF in the Czech Republic and so we wanted to choose a name that originated from there. With this response, he instantly looked incredibly embarrassed and responded with an apology saying "I'm so sorry for prying".

Even though I'd quite happily and freely provided this information, I was met by the expectation that I might have been embarrassed by the question. This spoke volumes to me about the stigma that still surrounds assisted conception. Of course, I didn't think he had over-stepped the mark in the slightest by asking about the origin of my daughter's name!

I am sure his reaction was partly a generational one, but it still shocked me. It was probably best that I didn't also mention that she was here all thanks to egg donation; that would have probably floored him! No wonder so many of us don't feel comfortable to open up about something such as IVF when it still seems like such an alien concept to some.

That's why I'm so passionate about raising awareness and starting these much-needed conversations, and I encourage others to do the same. It's only by doing this that we can lose the taboo surrounding infertility – needing a little help from science is nothing to be embarrassed about!

Becky Kearns @definingmum

Please don't...

Now, that I'm telling you I'm dealing with infertility, please don't try and 'fix it' for me. You can't. Trust me. Please, don't say 'I read an article about ....' Or 'My neighbours boss's sister-in-law's best friend tried for ten years and then went on holiday......' because that makes me feel worse. Please, don't pity me or look at me with sad eyes. Please, don't tell me about a celebrity who's just had a baby and start talking about them – this won't take my mind off the fact that I don't have a baby.

You could, instead, ask me "How are you?" and wait to hear my answer. You could say "I'm here for you."

Take my lead – if I'm not talking about it, then at that moment, I'm fine, so please, don't remind me by asking me questions. If I do start talking about how unfair it is, then it would really help me if you just listened.

Sheila @fertilitybooks

From the 'Think! What Not To Say' campaign videos

"Everything happens for a reason"

No. Just no. This is not helpful if someone is grieving a failed cycle or a miscarriage. Try to respect what that person is going through and understand that they need validation, not throw away comments, however well intentioned.

#humourandcompassion

Alice Rose @thisisalicerose

From the blog: Ten ways to save your marriage during infertility

Infertility poses a formidable challenge to even the strongest of marriages. First, there is the disappointment of learning that you and your soulmate are not exactly naturals at this procreation thing. Add testing, scheduled sex, and hormone-infused treatment to your relationship, along with a period of waiting and hoping, and then just a plain old period. Sprinkle in a recurring cycle of grief and a dash of doubt and you are on the fast track to isolation … the number one marriage killer.

Let's be clear. As much as you yearn for a child, your marriage must continue to take priority. No couple wants their long-awaited baby to arrive to a mommy and daddy on the brink of divorce. Yet, the arduous task of achieving pregnancy can cause couples to lose sight of their love for each other.

My marriage survived, despite a shortage of helpful guidance at the time. I wish my husband and I had had a TTC guru to guide us on what to do, to keep our relationship from resembling an episode of *Marriage Boot Camp*. So, here's me, a 10-year infertility survivor, suggesting what you should do.

1. Date

Remember, how much fun you and your husband/partner had when you first met? You probably had a romantic playlist, a favorite restaurant, and even a secret language. Marriages undergoing chronic infertility need a weekly dose of fun, whether frugal or frivolous.

2. Make love (not babies)

We infertiles know all about babymaking sex. The kind of sex that is scheduled with painstaking accuracy and ends with hips propped up on pillows. For those who are TTC, babymaking often overshadows lovemaking, but it doesn't have to be so. Break out the candles, crank up the Barry White and pour the wine. Leave the ratty t-shirt and elastic-waist jammie pants in the drawer and slip on something pretty. Need some inspiration? Read: *Song of Songs*, the raciest book in the Bible, and remember: God inspired Solomon to pen those steamy verses!

3. Get away

When a Pottery Barn store full of candles isn't enough to light the fire in a bedroom filled with regret, it's time to get away. Be it, Bed and Breakfast or Holiday Inn Express, the investment in your marriage is worth the cash you're able to sink into it. Sometimes, simply placing yourselves in a new environment with new possibilities hits the reset button and allows for a fresh perspective (read: romance).

4. **Take up a new hobby**

Have you ever tried rock climbing? Glamping? How about modelling clay on a potter's wheel or Renaissance re-enactment? Now is the time to summon your inner adventurer. Trying out a new skill or hobby will allow you to take a break from infertility and focus on a vital aspect of bonding ... fun.

5. **Send love notes**

Writing — or even texting — a note to your husband/ partner shows that you think about him even when you're not together. Be specific. Tell him what you appreciate about him and why you still choose to be with him now, even in the midst of your infertility struggle.

6. **Limit infertility talk**

You know the neighbor who blathers on about her bunions? The co-worker who complains daily about the newest directive from your boss? You're not likely to invite these Debbie Downers into your kitchen for a cup of tea. Constant talk of infertility treatment and grief puts the same damper on a marital relationship.

While planning and scheduling are a necessary part of TTC, don't allow this discussion to overshadow the blessings you both found in your life together. The plan? Treat the topic of infertility like an agenda item at a business meeting. Handle necessary discussions for the day, check it off your list, and move on. Then plop down on the couch in front of a favorite sitcom or romcom and engage in some endorphin-producing belly laughter. Infertility specialists would do well to prescribe an hour daily of lighthearted Netflix viewing.

7. **Hold hands**

Often infertility causes us to skip past some of the best

parts of bonding with our spouse. After all, when the goal is making a baby, what's the point of foreplay? As it turns out, plenty. Taking time to physically connect with your spouse, beyond intercourse, will bond you emotionally and create an irreplaceable companionship absent in any other relationship. And while you're holding hands, don't miss other points of connection such as eye to eye and voice to voice. Want to know more about the importance of daily bonding? Google it.

8. **Kiss deeply**

Kissing is another aspect of the marital relationship that often gets left in the dust when chasing after a positive pregnancy test. If you ditched making out somewhere along Infertility Road, pick it up, dust it off, and take it for another spin. Kissing allows couples to communicate deeply without words. The message? I cherish you, and you alone.

9. **Worship**

Infertility causes us to hyper-focus on what we have lost. Worship redirects our attention to what cannot be taken away, namely a God we can trust who works out every detail of our story for our good. Attending church together will help you and your spouse reaffirm your commitment to God and to each other at a time when life often feels like it's falling apart.

10. **Connect with other infertile couples**

Do you ever get tired of the clueless world shoving their pregnancy progress and baby photos in your face? Enter people who've been there. Hanging with another infertile couple is like being wrapped in a fuzzy blanket of comfort and mutual understanding. Befriend at least one couple that's on your wavelength and prepare to let down your guard. In this season of waiting, you need friends who get you, no explanation needed.

What if, as you pursue adding a child to your family, you continued to pursue your spouse as well? Doing so honors your first commitment and prepares you and your husband, not only for a child, but for a lifetime of loving each other well. Taking small steps each day will ensure that your marriage stays on track during infertility. Making these ten marriage-builders a habit will prepare you and your spouse to face infertility — and parenting — together.

Sarah Rollandini @ infertility_cheerleader

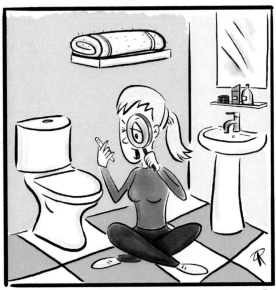

"I can definitely see a 2nd pink line"

Be there, listen and ask

I would have been due this week. Not a day goes by that I don't think of it. The miscarriage we had, the baby we lost, the infertility we're facing, and the way I thought things *should* be by now. For many people having a baby is a choice, but for those of us who can't 'decide and do', our choice becomes an expensive, exhausting mission. A mission we'd never choose to be on and one we can't escape from.

Infertility is all encompassing. My husband and I have been trying to conceive for over three years, with an 'if it happens it happens' attitude for at least three years prior to that. I never believed we'd be here. I didn't think it would happen to us. I know that may sound arrogant, and to some degree it is. You see, I've been with him since I was fifteen years old. I'm thirty-one now and have been dreaming of our babies since Freshman year of college. To say we've been waiting a lifetime would be an understatement. To say that every month that passes and my period shows is not more gut-wrenching than the last, would be a lie. To say that with every pregnancy announcement, every beautiful growing belly and baby I pass on the street, my entire self-weakens, would be truer than the faint of heart could ever handle.

My advice to anyone who loves someone who is suffering infertility is to be there, listen and ask. Be there during the important dates: the procedures, the would-have-been-due-dates, the results, the good news and the bad. Listen, when they choose to share with you. Resist the urge to compare them to someone you know, or something you heard, and be there for them in their specific situation. They will appreciate it more than you know. And lastly, don't be afraid to ask. Ask how they're doing. Ask if there's anything you can do to help. Ask them to brunch, or a pedicure, or a movie: anything that will help distract their worried mind for a brief moment in time.

Infertility is a lonely roller coaster with two passengers. Be there to fill up the seats.

Amelia Freeman @infertilityblows

Pregnancy announcements

Pregnancy announcements are really difficult for us to deal with in real life, on Instagram and Facebook. It's even difficult seeing pregnancy announcements from people you don't know. I can remember Prince Harry announcing his wife's pregnancy soon after getting married, and I was affected by that.

Most of our friends have had their children now so there aren't many pregnancy announcements for us to deal with. But when we do have them, it's extremely upsetting, as you end up feeling guilty, because your first thoughts aren't of happiness for the person making the announcement. In my case, I'm usually upset and angry because of my own situation. I think my wife's the stronger one. I know she's upset when pregnancies get announced, but she can be happy for them, whereas I still find it hard, so I'm still having counselling to try and help me deal with the anger.

Gareth James, UK

From the 'Think! What Not To Say' campaign videos

"Some people are just not that fertile"

Oh, are they meant to nod and say: "Thank you so much for that, I feel so much better now about the fact that we can't have children!"

#humourandcompassion

Alice Rose @thisisalicerose

Things infertile women want women with children to know

With one in seven couples going through infertility, it's very likely that you know a woman who is – it could be your sister, cousin, aunt, friend, colleague or neighbour. Infertility doesn't care whether the woman is rich or not, what her skin colour is, whether she went to uni, whether she drinks or not – it affects anyone. Many suffer in silence and keep their infertility private, whilst others are open and talk freely. Just like the differences in women, so are the causes of infertility, and it's as likely to be a male factor as it is female. Here are what we would like to share with our friends who have children and haven't experienced infertility. Thank you for reading.

1. We are jealous of you – we don't mean to be, but we just can't help it, and we don't want to admit it, but it's true. We're not jealous all the time, just some of the time. This is not the same as hating you, definitely not. We're jealous because you have what we desperately want and don't know if we will ever have it. We see the joy and happiness children bring you and we want nothing more than to experience that too. We would cut off our right arm to know what it's like to be a Mum.

2. This brings me to the subject of baby showers – please don't be upset that I may decline and if I do, you and the other guests will be thankful that gloomy-pants-I-may-just-burst-into-tears isn't there. I am truly happy for you and love that you are pregnant, but see the above explanation, and forgive me.

3. Even though we can be jealous some of the time and politely decline baby showers, we do still very much want to be friends – we have a history, we know things about each other that others don't know; we have a bond. But while I'm coping with infertility, I have to put myself first and look after me. I do want to remain

involved in your life and your children's lives, so please don't exclude me from celebrations and special events, as that makes me feel even more isolated. I'm sorry if sometimes you feel awkward around me; I will be open with you, but you must promise to be open with me too. Hopefully it won't be for long and the normal me will be back again, very soon.

4. Acts of kindness, texts, messages, cards are appreciated more than you will ever know – especially on days like Mother's Day, because everything about this day reminds us of what we aren't. However, we live with infertility every day, and every day, we hurt at some point, so thoughtful touches can make the difference between us having a crap day and having a good day.

5. Please don't give us advice on how to get pregnant – it's kind of you to care, but trust me, when I say we have read, heard and tried everything already. Saying this makes us want to beat you around the head with something big and heavy. Sorry, we have researched and read more than is decent. When you hear a piece of research about the latest super-food, trust me, I've already heard about it on one of the many infertility groups/forums I'm on. It's old news. When you think, I'll be interested to hear what the cashiers-aunts-best-friends-neighbour did and got pregnant, we are not the same person and there are hundreds of causes of infertility. Plus, I'm trying to get pregnant with a different man.

6. Please don't tell me to 'just adopt' – there is nothing 'just' about adopting. Like you, I would like to get pregnant and have my own baby. I haven't chosen infertility and I want to be pregnant and have a baby. It may take a lot of help from science and the medical world, but I still have hope. Infertility isn't easy and adoption isn't easy either. In some countries it costs thousands. In all countries it costs emotionally, as adoption doesn't erase the pain of infertility.

7. I'm really sorry, but I can't empathise with you when you complain about pregnancy, motherhood or your children – because I am jealous of all these three things. Every infertile woman has made a promise to herself that should she get pregnant and become a Mum, she will try so hard never to complain, because she wants this miracle every second of every day – remember, we'll cut off our right arm. To us it feels like you are taking these miracles for granted and we can't relate to that. Before you get angry at us, we do understand that motherhood is hard and that some people have a pregnancy that makes them feel sick, so we aren't expecting perfection. What I'm saying is that we can't relate to why you would complain about pregnancy and children when we want it so badly, in the same way that you can't relate to never experiencing a pregnancy, or ever having a child.

Sheila @fertilitybooks

Bubble of peace

There's a lot of things that can upset you when you're trying to conceive (TTC), isn't there?

Whilst this may feel hard to take control of, there is something that can help: your Bubble of Peace. For it to work, you need to understand what's going on in your head. When it comes to emotional pain, it isn't what we experience that hurts, but the meaning we give to that experience. Before infertility, the things that hurt now, probably, didn't hold much meaning in the past – such as, a pregnant woman walking down the street, or a mother holding her new-born baby. Seeing a pregnant woman, or a new mother, for example, can represent the loss of what you don't have, hence the difficult feelings.

Without any conscious effort. the chatter begins in your head; "Not another pregnant woman, why do I keep seeing them? It isn't fair. Everyone else can get pregnant easily, why can't I? I'm never going to get pregnant". This is where the Bubble of Peace helps you choose what you take notice of. Your mind is powerful, so all you have to do is imagine that you are stepping inside a bubble, much like the ones you make when you blow through a bubble hoop, but bigger and stronger.

Once inside your bubble, take your mind back to the most peaceful time in your life, when you felt calm, confident, happy and enjoying life. You can also fill it with your strengths — if you doubt you have them, take notice of how you manage to get up and get through each day, despite the intense emotional pain you are going through.

Any time you are feeling that life is too much, imagine stepping into that bubble and surround yourself with all of those wonderful feelings. Your subconscious mind doesn't know the difference between real and imagined events, so the more vividly you tap into the events that you've stored in your Bubble of Peace, the better the experience you will have whilst you're in there.

It might take some strength to take the first step inside, but once you get accustomed to utilising your Bubble of Peace, you'll be amazed just how much you are the one in control of how you feel and think, rather than allowing external factors to swamp you with feelings of despair.

Dany Griffiths @freedomfertilityformula

TTC in a bigger body

When you want to get pregnant in a larger body, you will likely be told that you need to lose weight to improve your fertility and to access any support from your healthcare professionals. We are led to believe that it is all our fault that we are unable to get pregnant, and that if we could simply lose some weight, we would get pregnant easily.

This is not true. Research now suggests that intentional weight loss is far more damaging to our health than getting pregnant in a larger body. It's not the fat that causes the increased health risks we see in bigger bodies, but the restrictive and unhealthy diets that we feel forced to try repeatedly, and the discrimination we face in our daily lives from healthcare professionals, because of our size.

There are doctors and other healthcare professionals that will support you and not judge you or shame you. Find them and get the support you rightly deserve as you prepare for pregnancy. Learning how to advocate for your body and your health isn't something that we should have to do, but it's something we need to do in our society right now to get access to the tests and treatments that will most support our health.

If you've been on the dieting train for a while now, intellectually, you know that it never works. You may lose some weight at the start, but it always comes back. It's not because you are doing it wrong or that you aren't good enough. It's because diets don't work. It's not that you haven't found the 'right diet' yet, but because any form of restrictive eating will only work in the short term.

So, what can you do right now to support your health and move away from focusing on weight loss?

Explore what it feels like to trust your body again. If you need some direction, look up 'Intuitive Eating' and start with the ten basic principles. Learning how to trust your body and listen to its cues is the most powerful way to improve your health and fertility.

The biggest step you can take is to believe that your body is capable of having a healthy pregnancy right now, not when you weigh less.

Nicola Salmon @fatpositivefertility

Primary and secondary infertility – the same but different

I've had two difficult fertility journeys; the first took two and a half years – not a long time compared to others, but it felt long enough. A year in, I suffered an early miscarriage, which completely broke me. Personally, I didn't feel I had lost a person or a baby, but the dream, the future, and the family I so desperately wanted. Each month got harder and harder, the hope leading to disappointment, and the pain which was hidden from friends, family and work.

It took over my life, caused stress in my relationship with the focus on timing, tracking my cycle, temperature, ovulation, and then the hell of the two-week wait. Am I, aren't I? Do I test early or wait? What alternative therapy should I try next? Will it work?

I came off social media, because it was too painful to see everyone else, (seemingly), getting pregnant easily and enjoying their perfect family life.

We had unexplained infertility, and I now feel like my subconscious was protecting me from the emotional pain of my miscarriage, by preventing another pregnancy. Only when I addressed these emotional issues did I fall pregnant again.

After having my son, I fell pregnant again quickly. I couldn't believe how easy pregnancy could be. But something didn't feel right. I was told that all pregnancies are different, so I tried to focus on that. At my twelve-week scan, I found out I'd miscarried, which was devastating. Then we were back to that more familiar feeling and getting pregnant became difficult and stressful for us. I learned so much from this about instinct, and the difference between worrying that something is wrong and having a feeling that something is wrong.

Secondary infertility was really different; it wasn't possible to avoid children and families as I had to take my son to playgroups or to the park. My new fixation was on age gaps, calculating it each month and trying to work out the age difference between other people's children. Then all my friends were announcing their pregnancies and having their second babies while we were still trying. It definitely impacted those relationships, as I didn't want to hear how tiring it was to be pregnant and look after a toddler, or how much more stressful it was having two children, compared to one.

Now I can look back on both these experiences and recognise that I am stronger for it. I don't know what kind of mother I would have been without this struggle, but I feel grateful every day for having my son and being pregnant again.

Having lived in secrecy about trying for a baby for so long, after having my son it was amazing speaking to other mums who'd also had a difficult journey to motherhood. We were now free to talk about it as we'd finally made it to the other side. I immediately felt a connection to these mums; not that our experiences were the same, but that we knew how hard this journey is that many, simply, don't understand.

Nicola Headley @nicola_freedomfertility

Supporting male fertility

When a couple are having trouble getting pregnant, the focus often turns to a woman's health. But men can be contributors to fertility problems too. Experts are now saying that infertility is due to a male-factor issue approximately 40% of the time, so the mindset needs to change.

The good news is that certain dietary and lifestyle factors have been shown to support male fertility and improve chances of pregnancy. But this requires men to be proactive about their role in the fertility journey. Below are some basic tips that may help men support their fertility through diet and lifestyle changes:

1. Refrain from recreational drug use and tobacco products. The old saying that 'Everything is OK in moderation' does not apply to recreational drugs or tobacco when it comes to fertility. A growing body of evidence is supporting the recommendation to refrain from using any of these products when trying to conceive.

2. Tackle obesity, if a man is considered obese. In general, those who are considered obese are at a higher risk of having fertility challenges. If you have a body mass index (BMI) that is thirty or higher, you are considered obese. In a review of thirty studies that included over 115,000 men, researchers found the following results:

   - obesity was associated with more incidences of sperm with DNA fragmentation and abnormal shape (among other sperm-related issues)

   - the rate of live births per cycle of ART (Assisted Reproduction Technology) for obese men was reduced, compared with men who were not considered obese

   - the risk of a pregnancy resulting in miscarriage was

increased by 10% if the man was obese at the time of conception

- gradual weight loss to reach a desirable weight is recommended

3.   Follow a Mediterranean diet and lifestyle pattern. Adherence to the Mediterranean diet is significantly associated with higher sperm concentration, total sperm count, and sperm motility. Dietary patterns characterized by high intakes of fruit, vegetables, whole grains, fish and low intake of meats are associated with better semen quality, and may have more positive fertility-related symptoms.

A Mediterranean diet is a general term for a diet that many eat who live near the Mediterranean Sea. There are slight variations, but for medical purposes, certain guidelines remain consistent.

Below are the basic principles of the Mediterranean diet:

- high consumption of fruits, vegetables, whole-grain bread and other cereals such as beans, nuts and seeds

- olive oil is an important monounsaturated fat source

- fish and seafood are consumed at least two times a week

- dairy products and poultry are consumed in low to moderate amounts

- eggs are consumed zero to four times a week

- red meat and sweets are rarely eaten

4.   Enjoy a daily handful of nuts, or two. Nuts, such as walnuts, almonds and hazelnuts, are rich in fertility

nutrients, including plant protein, omega-3s and antioxidants. Research suggests that nuts may boost male fertility by improving sperm fertility indicators such as improved sperm count.

5.   Limit or cut out processed meats which can interfere with male fertility, <u>according to research.</u>[1]

- Replacing processed meats with poultry or fish <u>may boost fertility</u> [2]

- Processed meats to avoid or minimize include bacon, sausage, ham, corned beef, beef jerky and salami

These tips are a great starting-point for men to get their bodies "fertility-ready". Incorporating these diet and lifestyle choices will be a wonderful way to support male fertility.

Lauren Manaker @LaurenManaker_RDN.

1. https://www.ncbi.nlm.nih.gov/pubmed/26206344
2. https://www.ncbi.nlm.nih.gov/pubmed/24850626

From the 'Think! What Not To Say' campaign videos

"Don't leave it too long, because otherwise the age gap will be too big!"

They're trying! They're aware. Gentle respect …

#humourandcompassion

Alice Rose @thisisalicerose

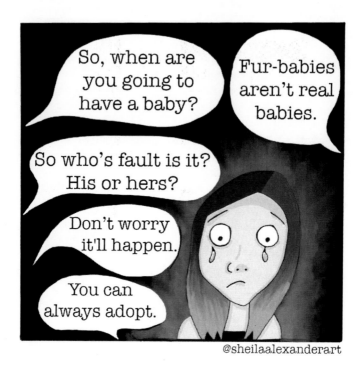

@sheilaalexanderart

Letter to my infertile partner

Having sex is fun, right? It certainly is until you start trying to conceive without success. As the months roll on, sex becomes less about pleasure and intimacy and more about the task at hand. It becomes timed, regimented. "Just come in me, make it quick", she said. And then finally, sex becomes sad. It's a reminder of what you are failing to achieve.

Getting the romance and intimacy back after an infertility diagnosis is not an easy feat. It's a dark and tiring road, leaving you feeling hopeless. But as long as you continue to reinforce your partner in a positive way, it is possible to get things back on track.

To my Infertile Partner

It's not your fault. Stop reflecting on every single life decision you made and wondering what you could have done differently. Watching you beat yourself up about this breaks my heart. We are a team. This isn't you versus me. As a couple we are infertile, and we will figure this out together.

I am not going to leave you. I would not be better off with someone else. Stop saying that. There is no one else I want to share my life with and build a family with. I chose you for your humor, kind heart and work ethic. I chose you for so much more than your fertility.

I am still attracted to you. You are just as beautiful as the day I met you, and a little bit more each day. I am so proud to call you mine. Yours is still the only smile I see in the room.

I want sex to be fun again. I want to see your confidence back in the bedroom. Your mojo is not lost, it just went away for a while. I want the laughter and the pillow talk. I want to have sex at all times of the month again, not just near ovulation day. Let's be spontaneous and curious and playful, the way we used to be, without pressure.

We will have a family, no matter what it takes. We are partners. We promised ourselves to one another through the good and the bad, and I will always honor that. We can conquer anything as long as we're together.

Love,

Your Fertile Partner

@HerFertilityDiary

These feelings are completely normal

'Trying to Conceive' – three short, simple words that hold so much significance for so many, and for us as a couple, have come to shape and define most of the past nineteen months. We started 'TTC' on our wedding night. I was thirty-six and my husband thirty-two. In reality, I'd been 'ready' to become a mother long before then, but my husband didn't have the same urgency to begin parenthood, coupled with us becoming wrapped up in wedding planning, we decided to wait until after our 'big day' to start our family. Having bought my dress twelve months before our actual wedding, I'd also decided that it wouldn't accommodate a bump of any kind, so a baby would have to wait a little longer. The irony that a large bump is the only thing I want to be parading right now doesn't escape me, and I can't help but wish we'd started trying to conceive sooner.

One of the things I've struggled with the most in learning to accept my infertility is how it has made me question, and reassess parts of my life, as well as doubt past decisions I've made. I now feel in a constant rush against time to get pregnant and would love nothing more than to rewind that biological clock. But what I've also realised is that infertility is unpredictable and unfair. No one can plan or prepare for it.

I'd always been aware that there was a possibility my fertility had been affected by the gruelling eight months of chemo I'd had at the age of twenty-six, but I'd been lucky enough to preserve ten eggs prior to starting my treatment, which I'd banked purely as an insurance policy as I'd never considered that one day I'd need to use them. Even though I'd had cancer twice before the age of thirty, my cycle had returned shortly after finishing treatment and an ultrasound scan had shown my ovaries appeared 'normal' a few months before we married. Plus, two friends who'd had the same type of cancer had both gone on to have healthy pregnancies, one of them falling pregnant the first month of trying, so I was hopeful and positive it would happen for us some time soon. I also naively told myself that I couldn't be THAT unlucky to have had cancer AND be infertile; surely life wouldn't be that cruel — but I was, and it is. Just like a cancer diagnosis, infertility is ruthlessly unfair and indiscriminate.

I recall the first few months we tried to conceive as being an exciting and optimistic time — each month wondering if this would be 'the one' when we got our positive test. In the end I didn't ever need to do a test, because right on time, if not a little early, my period ALWAYS arrived. In May of that year, five months after we began TTC, I was convinced I was pregnant. My breasts were sore and swollen and I was certain that I felt 'different'. When my period arrived a couple of days later, I remember feeling sad and frustrated for the first time, finally wondering when our time would arrive. At this point we changed supplements, both cut out all alcohol, reduced caffeine, and became a little more 'serious' in our mission to conceive; albeit losing some of the 'fun' in the process.

Summer 2017, brought an unexpected pregnancy announcement from my sister-in-law and despite feeling happy for my brother and his wife and excited at the prospect of becoming an aunty, the TTC jealousy monster reared its ugly head, and I experienced pangs of resentment and thoughts of unfairness that it wasn't us sharing such joyous news when we'd been 'trying' for longer. These feelings, I've realized, are completely natural during our relentless process of TTC, however unhelpful and unhealthy they might be. I've learnt to let them wash over me and not feel guilty for having them. Infertility is brutal and all consuming, and we have enough to worry about without beating ourselves up about feelings that are completely normal — we're all human after all. I just have to keep telling myself that one day our time will come and one way or another, we will become parents, because there are ALWAYS options out there, and seeking support from others also in the TTC community has helped me to feel a little less alone.

September 2018, delivered the results of the dreaded AMH test and the realisation that we were unlikely to conceive naturally. Much like my cancer diagnosis, it came as a thunderbolt and left me feeling devastated, numb and scared about the future.

We're now nearly two years down the line since we started TTC and so much has happened, although little has changed. We've experienced a heart-breaking miscarriage, a cancelled IVF cycle, and a whole load of other unexpected challenges and upset. I've been open and honest about my infertility and started an Instagram account to connect with other couples in a similar position. The TTC online community has brought me unexpected friendships and solidarity from people who know exactly how I'm feeling. Just like the cancer community, I also reluctantly joined all those years ago, and am still very much involved with, the TTC community has led me to some of the kindest souls who have provided strength and comfort during the darkest of times, and also the hope to continue as we embark upon cycle two of IVF.

@eggainst_the_odds

From the 'Think! What Not To Say' campaign videos

"I know EXACTLY how you feel. I was devastated every time it didn't work for THREE MONTHS when we were trying."

Trying for three months and going through years and years of treatment is not the same thing. Don't try and 'understand' if you haven't been through it. Even if you have, our experiences are so unique, so try to respect every story's complexities.

#humourandcompassion

Alice Rose @thisisalicerose

An excerpt from the book 'Warrior'

I spent two and a half years of my life struggling to manage my obsession with getting pregnant. It affected my whole life in ways I would never have anticipated. Trying to conceive, for good or bad, became my sole purpose. When I was standing in the queue in a coffee shop, my mind would be going over dates and calculations, working out the optimum time to have sex. When I was in a meeting at work, I would be arguing with myself about whether to take a pregnancy test a day earlier than I'd allowed myself to. On the train home, I was wondering whether I should have done that shoulder stand for an extra two minutes, as that could have been the *one thing* that made the difference between my dreams coming true and trudging on in this state of semi-existence.

The trying/struggling to conceive journey can be a lonely and isolating place. It's not easy to talk about — people don't know what to say. If you're a stressed-out parent with a toddler who's causing havoc in a supermarket, you can exchange wry smiles with other parents — the older generation who've been there, or basically anybody else who happens to be around.

Being a parent is hard work, but feeling frustrated because your child won't put down the bag of sweets and move on to the shampoo aisle, or being exasperated because your child has thrown their food all over the floor (again), are actually *good problems* to have. I say this because they're relatable. You can use them to bond with others, they make good anecdotes, and you know that however annoying these things are at the time, you're blessed to be experiencing them.

Infertility is a *bad problem* to have. When you're self-consciously brushing tears from your cheeks, overcome with emotion in the nappy aisle, there's nobody there rolling their eyes with you or offering an understanding smile. When you have to leave the room because someone has announced their pregnancy and they've only been trying a couple of months, you're pulling yourself together alone in the toilets. This doesn't make an amusing anecdote over dinner with friends, later. It makes people uncomfortable. I want to change that. I want it to be okay to say "Hey, I'm struggling to get pregnant, and it's tough" — and for people to know what to say back.

Tori Day – author

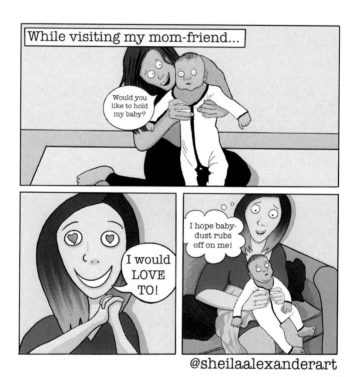

@sheilaalexanderart

I told my friends

Should I tell my friends that I have a poor semen analysis? OK guys, I'm not going to give too much advice on this, but what I will say is that I did tell most people that we were trying to conceive. And anyone that was not supportive, I simply don't speak to anymore. For me, it felt better to get it off my chest rather than bundle it up! It's your call, but that's my story.

@the.swim.team

From the blog: Where to get the support you need during the holiday season

It's that time of year again, folks: the holiday season. Also known as 'The emotional minefield'. The holidays can be challenging when you're on a fertility journey. While you might feel alone, sad, angry, bitter, despondent or in despair about your experiences throughout the year, these feelings can be intensely magnified at this time.

You're triggered by virtually everything: seeing happy families and pregnant women everywhere, from your sister-in-law who's pregnant by accident with her fourth kid, to strangers with babies in the shopping mall. Mustering up fake holiday cheer at the office party you could care less about, because you'd rather have the job of Stay-At-Home Mom. Opening one more ornament given by a long-lost relative who means well, but doesn't know that the only thing you really wanted was two pink lines.

During this time, it's very important to make sure that you're able to tap into the emotional support you need. Because you *will* need it. Emotional support is paramount on the fertility journey. A national study conducted by RESOLVE in the United States found that coping with emotional challenges during fertility treatment is one of the biggest hurdles a patient goes through, and can be a significant factor to a patient dropping out of treatment. Put simply, the physical toll of fertility treatment can be a walk in the park compared to the emotional effects this journey can have. So, it's important to be cognizant of your emotional needs during fertility; even more so on the holidays. You're just so much more fragile at this time of year.

It can be hard to know where to turn when you need emotional support, especially if you haven't thought about it in advance. I strongly recommend you do think about it in advance, and have a few ideas in your back pocket, so that when the time comes, you're ready for it.

Here are a few suggestions on resources to tap into for emotional support:

Support Groups

You can attend an in-person support group, be part of an online support group, or both. Both offer distinct advantages. In-person groups obviously give you the benefit of connecting in-person with the group leader and other members of the group. Being around other people, especially people who understand what you're going through, because they're going through it themselves, can help you feel less alone or isolated. Many fertility clinics offer support groups for their patients.

Online support groups

If you feel a little shy in groups or more reluctant to make an in-person connection, online support groups can offer you a more private connection while still giving you the support you need. Most online groups are closed, whereby only the members of the group can see the discussions taking place, making the online group a safe space to share.

Another awesome thing about online support groups is that they transcend space and time, and you can connect with like-minded women from all over the world. My online group, 'Path to Your Fertile Self', brings together members from at least ten different countries on six continents. These are women that would never have the opportunity to meet were it not for the wonderful technology of the Internet.

Your fertility Nurse

If support groups aren't your thing, you can find support in other places. If you're doing fertility treatment, your fertility nurse is a valuable resource. Do not overlook your nurse! She's there to help you and make your journey less stressful. Not only does she guide you through the treatment process, she's there to answer all of your questions and can be a rock of support.

Fertility Coaches

Like myself, a fertility coach focuses on helping clients develop and achieve goals related to their fertility, health and wellness, and incorporate emotional support into their practice. Often, my clients show up for a session with a need to talk about their feelings towards their journey, rather than focus on whatever topic had been on the agenda for that day. And that's okay. We're trained to give clients what they need, when they need it.

Mental Health Professionals

There's a fine line, however, between coaching and therapy, and if I feel a client needs more than I'm qualified to give in terms of emotional support, I'll encourage her to see a therapist. Many therapists focus their practice on grappling with fertility challenges and may have even been through their own fertility journey.

Other wellness practitioners

Finally, many fertility clients take advantage of the power of different healing modalities to improve their fertility. Modality practitioners – including acupuncturists, massage therapists, Reiki practitioners, or reflexologists – often provide emotional support to their clients.

Stephanie Roth, @yourfertileself

Keep it simple

At what stage do you tell people you're trying to conceive? Who do you tell about your journey? How do you stay in touch with friends who are getting on with their lives, having babies, when you're facing a diagnosis of infertility?

Fiona, a client of mine, tearfully revealed to me how much she was dreading a pending girly spa weekend away. Usually she'd be counting the days until the get together, but this time was different. The pressure of infertility was overwhelming. Her friends didn't know about her upcoming IVF and she feared a reveal would ruin the fun for everyone. Would they treat her as a failure, ply her with advice and make her the centre of attention, for all the wrong reasons?

I asked her how she'd told her parents and family. "Very simply", she replied. "I just explained that David and I needed a bit of extra medical help to get pregnant, and that I'd need a bit of support, but nothing too over-the-top, like daily bulletins! I guess it's more of a 'watch this space' type of thing. To be honest, I don't know how I'll feel or what I'll need, so I'll have to play it by ear, as you say."

Keeping infertility or IVF announcements brief and simple allows people time to grasp your message. This goes for family, friends, employers, HR departments, bosses and work colleagues where appropriate. Be clear in your intention for the conversation, take control and guide the conversation.

With friends you might want to go further to explain your feelings — uncertainty about what you'll need, how you'd like to stay in touch, that treatment can take up a lot of time and energy, and that you might not be your usual sunny self while on meds — all of this, while not making everything about your journey.

Fiona told her girlfriends soon after they met at the hotel, before the weekend officially got going. Reactions to her news were varied and mostly positive. She was clear in her initial message that it was not clouding the weekend. "They were great and positive,' she told me later. "I timed it perfectly and then we moved onto the main business in hand at that moment – dinner!"

Even if you handpick your supporters, they may find it hard to step up and support you in just the way you need. Mindreading is an inexact skill at the best of times, so some Google mapping makes it easier for everybody to be in the right place for you. If your tribe gets the right guidelines, they'll enjoy showing up for you.

Infertility is isolating and that only adds to the distress of infertility and IVF struggles, so it's worth making the effort it takes to stay in touch with family and friends. Online chats are great, anonymous forums may help but they lack the warmth and connection a meet-up delivers. A quick text may be all you can deal with, and sometimes a call says more if you're not in the space for meeting up.

Coffee and lunch dates are great ways to connect, stay in touch, even have a laugh to get a reprieve from the relentless grind. Crucially, they're in a neutral space and are time limited. If that sounds a bit paranoid, let me explain why it's good. If you visit someone's home it's more intimate, the spotlight is on you, and there's no real timeframe set. In a café setting you're on a more level conversational playing field, with a natural timeline. Conversation flows with less risk of feeling overwhelmed, keeping you connected and in the loop.

And when someone shares this news with you, remember that it's about them, and not you. So, there's no need for advice, opinions or anecdotes. Simply listen, hear the news, and ask what is expected of you. The main thing is to let the folk who matter know how you'd like them to react to your news, how to stay in touch and how to support you best.

Helena Tubridy @helenatubridy

"Do you think you should try losing a few pounds because you are a bit ... overweight?"

This isn't supportive! Just be supportive!

#humourandcompassion

Alice Rose @thisisalicerose

Write a letter you never send

Maintaining relationships when you're struggling to conceive can be fraught with those awful 'I'm-so-happy-for-you' through tears of frustration moments. It can be tempting to just throw your social life out the window when your focus is on adding to your family. But you're going to need a close network of people in your life to help you get through it all.

Even though it will be tough, I urge you to be that friend that shows up to other friend's baby showers. At times, it will hurt like hell, and you'll have to reapply your make up after an ugly cry in the car two streets away from the party. #beenthere. It hurts to hear how happy your friend is, or how they weren't even really trying, or "gee, I just want this to be over..." but that is a strength you have to find when things aren't happening to schedule. I've felt it. Sometimes though, people are just plain thoughtless. Other times, they just don't get what you're going through.

It took IVF (in-vitro fertilisation) for us to have kids, after years with no 'accidents' and a couple of failed inseminations (IUIs). We lost our first IVF baby at seven weeks, after being incredibly ill for much of the pregnancy. Then some of our dearest friends announced they were pregnant. I was in bits. We had been friends forever, and I knew she'd struggled to conceive too, but

I was devastated. And I knew my attitude sucked. Who was I to be upset at this beautiful news?

So, I wrote her a letter that was never meant to be sent. In it, I told her that I was proud of her and truly glad for her. But I also needed to express that I was at the same time heartbroken that I couldn't say that I was pregnant too. It was a way of getting all of the hurt and the 'poor me' thoughts out of my head. Things that I never would have wanted to say to her in person. That way, I could focus on the next step, keep going, and no longer feel the need to clap my hand over my mouth to prevent mis-speaking in front of them. I was never going to send the letter, but I found the process of getting it out of my head truly healing, like lifting a weight off my shoulders.

Here's what I drafted:

Hi

I just wanted to address the elephant in the room and discuss something with you, so I don't give you the wrong impression or act weird and make you wonder whether you did something to upset me.

I love you both so very much and I can't possibly express how very happy I am for you to be pregnant - thrilled, relieved and proud for you doesn't begin to cover it.

But I am also ever so slightly envious... If things had gone differently, we would have had a "Me too!" moment at Christmas, as the timing of your good news could so easily have meant that we were pregnant at the same time.

So, your announcement was a reminder of what could have been, and in my head, I was doing stupid 'What if?' scenarios and calculations. It's something I'm working through and it's totally not your problem ;-)

I just need you to know that from time to time, I may get a bit teary and appear to be upset, but it's not at you. So, now that that is said, I can prepare to be the world's greatest Aunty ;-)

Always,

Sandi

So, this is how it felt for me, to wish nothing but happiness for our friends and be smiling for them on the outside, but crying on the inside. I wasn't a green-eyed monster, just a broken woman struggling with feeling left behind, as if I was failing to meet a basic expectation of me as a woman and a partner.

If you haven't experienced this situation yourself, I hope my sharing of this letter gives you some insight into why some people might not seem as happy about your baby news as you'd hoped. There are complicated emotions at play. Please, be understanding of the people in your life struggling with having to be patient about when, or if, they'll have kids.

If you've felt this situation yourself, I'm sorry that happened to you. It sucks. I'm sending you a hug. I want you to know that however you choose to deal with your grief is up to you, and everyone will find a personal way of healing in their own time. Perhaps writing letters you'll never send is something you might like to try out, to order your thoughts and process conflicted feelings. If someone hurts you with a question or an announcement, write it out. Tell them everything you wish you could say aloud and save it for later. It will lift some of the weight off your chest.

Sandi Friedlos @Sandifriedlos

Affirmations

An affirmation is a statement repeatedly said aloud to help you believe new information. Perhaps you learned your multiplication tables by repetition. Do you know the story of 'The Little Engine that Could' who kept saying "I think I can, I think I can" as he pulled a broken-down train over the mountain? Even though it was a struggle, he believed he could get over that mountain, and he did.

In the military, soldiers are not just strong physically but mentally as well. The ability to stay strong is not only in the body but in one's thoughts. They are taught to be mentally strong by repeatedly singing songs or learning how to respond to difficult challenges. When they meet a challenge on the battlefield, they automatically have the mindset to face and overcome the challenge.

When trying to conceive, people spend a lot of time focussing on the medical aspect of conception and can negate the mental and emotional aspect, which can have more ramifications than an impact to our physical body. As you begin investigative tests and treatments, your circumstances will start telling you this is not going to happen – you're too old, your cycles are irregular, his sperm aren't good swimmers. Your mind is fighting against this bombardment of information which is contrary to what you want.

Saying an affirmation aloud helps you to overcome the mental chatter of why this can't happen for you. Choose to believe differently than what your circumstances are telling you. The affirmation can also help you remain positive and hopeful.

To create your own affirmations, come up with a statement in the present tense that you choose to believe and write it down. Examples such as:

> I choose to believe that I ovulate each month
>
> I choose to believe I am fertile
>
> We choose to believe I'll have an easy conception, pregnancy, and birth.

Please be mindful of using future tense as this doesn't create the reality you want to attain. Your subconscious only understands the 'now' not past or future. A statement such as 'I will become pregnant' means that the event remains in the future and out of your reach. It's like saying "I'm going to Paris," which is the planning stage, rather than saying "I am enjoying being in Paris," which means you're already there. Affirmations must reflect what you desire as if it's already happening 'now'.

Using an affirmation means that you are deciding to create a new thought pattern so that you are able to override negative thoughts and beliefs with what it is you want to achieve. If you tell someone repeatedly that they are smart, they will eventually start believing it. The affirmation has the same effect and can be used for any situation, especially for the trying to conceive community.

Great affirmations to continually declare aloud:

- I choose to believe differently from what I've been told about my ability to conceive and have a healthy baby. I believe I will conceive and have a healthy, full-term baby.
- We choose to believe to have an easy conception, pregnancy and birth.
- I choose to believe my spouse/partner and I are healthy. Our reproductive systems work correctly, and at the right time, and produce perfectly formed eggs and sperm.
- I choose to believe it is right for me to have a child.

Salise Wright @Lohojo.uk

I should be able to cope

Something I'm always struck by when people seek counselling is how often they arrive with a sense of guilt that they 'should' be able to cope more effectively and that they don't really warrant a counselling session – and that's exactly how I felt when I arrived at my first counselling session, too!

Probably the most important thing for anyone in this situation to understand is that *everyone* finds infertility difficult, and that they are very much deserving of some additional support at this time.

When can counselling help?

You should be able to access counselling whenever you need it, whether that's before, during or after tests or treatment. There are a number of organisations that have counsellors who are specially trained in infertility, or you can search online, but ensure they are experienced with people going through infertility.

Sometimes people are worried about what counselling will entail. It really is *your* time to use exactly as you'd like, without any pressure from anything or anyone else.

Here are some of the ways that counselling can help when you're dealing with infertility:

- You can offload all the toxic emotions you've been carrying. All of those feelings that we try so hard to censor when we're with everyone else: the anger, the bitterness, the desperation, the envy, the grief, the guilt and the shame – they can all be shared, uncensored, with a fertility counsellor.
- You can talk freely in the knowledge that they won't be judging you, because they will understand that these feelings are a normal response to infertility. Be reassured that they will have supported many other women and men who have gone through the same emotions and issues as you.
- You can safely confront your fears. When trying to conceive is proving to be a struggle, anxious thoughts about when 'WILL I get pregnant' can overwhelm you. You might worry that you need IVF (in-vitro fertilisation), or what your future will look like if you don't have a baby. A counsellor won't offer you platitudes, but they will support you while you explore what lies beneath the fear, enabling you to identify what

matters to you and what you need to feel content with your life.

- You can get in touch with your hope. This may sound like a tall order, but often when we've been allowed to release and accept our fears along with other difficult emotions, our underlying strength starts to emerge.
- You can explore ways to manage the difficult relationships in your life and nurture the ones that give you strength – in a way that uniquely suits you and where you are in your life right now.
- You can take back some control. Infertility feels like a waiting game and so much of it is out of our control. Counselling can help you to make peace with the aspects of infertility that will always fall to chance, and to identify the choices that are still yours to make.
- You can just be you. Most important of all, you can take a break from needing to fit into any role of 'employee', 'partner', 'friend,' and be free to be yourself – whatever that looks like for you at the time of your counselling session. There are no expectations on you for that hour, which can come as a welcome relief during fertility treatment.

Rachel Cathan Author of *336 Hours*

From the 'Think! What Not To Say' campaign videos

"When we were trying to conceive, I had avocado every day, put my legs in the air after sex, and stayed really positive, so if you JUST do those three things..."

Dismisses the real and complex issues going through infertility presents; this isn't to say 'tips' can't potentially help, but your story is not their story and they've probably tried everything you can think of and more anyway! Utterly infuriating!

#humourandcompassion

Alice Rose @thisisalicerose

BFP?

I'd no idea what it meant, it's a mystery.

Like all the abbreviations are confusing, and the list is long.

I spent hours on the forum looking for a glossary, learning the language.

Talking to faceless friends through cyberspace, cycle buddies and forum mates.

Through a phrasebook of the unspeakable, with a language of its own.

B for Big

F for Fat

P for Positive

BFP

Big Fat Positive

How you eluded me and how you were missed from my forum signature.

Full of BFNs.

Big Fat Negatives.

Justine Bold @justine_bold

Negative Feelings

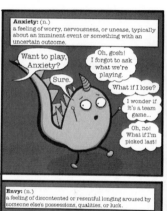

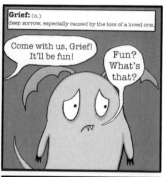

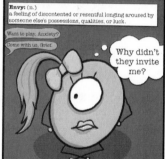

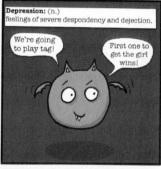

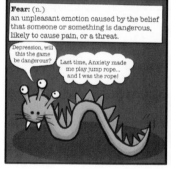

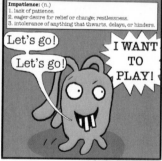

@sheilaalexanderart

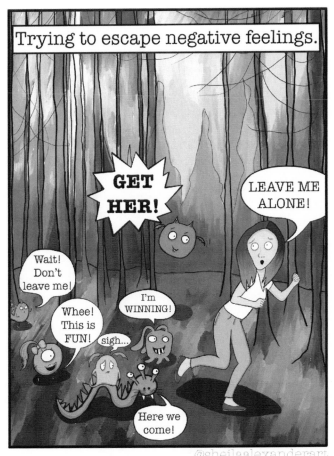

Take control of your fertility health

When I was about twenty-three my mum was diagnosed with an underactive thyroid which can be hereditary. When she told me her symptoms, I was sure I had it too. However, NHS tests with my GP said I was fine. I was offered antidepressants instead, which I refused as I wasn't depressed, just frustrated that I wasn't being listened to.

I started doing my own research and I KNEW my GP was wrong. I read how it would be almost impossible for a person with an untreated thyroid problem to get pregnant, and if by some miracle they did, to stay pregnant. As I was so young and nowhere near ready to start a family, fixing my fertility wasn't my main goal ... my overall health was.

I found a private doctor who confirmed that I had an underactive thyroid and advised that I would have to treat myself privately and self-medicate. Although an expensive route, I was prepared to do anything to be healthy. Over the years, more and more information and support became available, (I thank god for thyroid UK and it's forum), so I was able to have more affordable and therefore more regular blood testing which I did myself, and my medication was adjusted accordingly. I went back to my GP who was shocked at my private results, and agreed that, yes, there certainly was an issue with my thyroid. (I still self-medicate as lack of funding means the NHS are unable to give me the most important medication I need).

When I got to thirty-five years old and I was ready to become pregnant, all three of my babies were conceived on the first month of us trying.

By refusing to put my health solely into the hands of someone else, I changed my body from infertile to fertile, very quickly. Imagine if I had listened to them, I wouldn't have my beautiful babies today — a truly scary thought! I guess the moral of the story is trust your instincts, then do your own research so you can become your own health advocate. No one is going to care about your health and fertility more than you.

Please know that your GP only tests two or three of the eight things (listed below), that must be tested. For some, this will be enough. For others, like me, it isn't. Also, don't let them tell you your ranges are "normal". What they say is normal varies massively from GP to GP, and anyway normal isn't good enough; 'optimal' is what you need.

Keep printouts of your results and if you have an underactive thyroid, read the book *Your Healthy Pregnancy with Thyroid Disease* by D. Trentini and Mary Shomon to help you interpret your results.

1. TSH

2. T3

3. T4

4. Antibodies

5. Vit D

6. Vit B12

7. Folate

8. Ferritin

Eleanor Modral-Gibbons @fertility_manchester

Trying for a baby became more scientific

Like most married couples, we waited a few months to enjoy being married and then began thinking about starting a family. I specifically remember the first time we were officially 'trying'. We were so excited that we might make a baby. We were away at the time and kept wondering what our baby would look like and the names we liked and disliked. Unfortunately, a few weeks went by and I discovered I wasn't pregnant that month. We were disappointed, but knew it probably wouldn't happen the first month, so we continued trying, feeling hopeful. When month six ticked by, I remember starting to worry.

Almost everyone we knew got pregnant within the first month or two of trying, so we started to wonder if something was wrong. At that point I visited the GP who said that as I'd had issues with my cycle in the past, it would be worthwhile having some tests on both me and my husband to see what was happening. A few weeks later, we discovered that my husband's results were fine, but I was diagnosed with polycystic ovaries. We were told that it wouldn't be impossible for us to conceive naturally, but the likelihood was about 7%, and to give us the best chance we should have sex every couple of days. That was an enormous blow to us. When you are actually told what you were already thinking, it suddenly becomes more real. The realisation hit us that something so easy and natural may not happen for us. We knew that the act of trying for a baby would have to become more scientific and no longer romantic and this really affected our relationship. Sex just isn't fun when it's no longer spontaneous or planned out.

I remember thinking that if I were on a desert island with just the two of us, I could probably cope better with making a baby even if it took months or even years. Unfortunately, seeing colleagues and friends everyday who started looking at my tummy rather than my face when they said "hello", and analysing what I was eating and drinking just in case I was pregnant, made everything so much more difficult. I felt so much pressure to be pregnant and the fact that I didn't have a little bump made me feel incredibly insecure as if I was a failure. People were constantly asking if we were thinking about having children or had we started trying. These questions were so intrusive but, somehow, they seem to be socially acceptable questions to ask a woman who has just got married. During the first few months, it was easy to say "Oh no, not yet" or "We definitely do, but want to be married for a bit first," but later on the questions were met with tears from me and awkward silences from them.

After nine months of trying we decided that we'd tell family and close friends what the doctor had told us. Everyone was disappointed and felt sad for us. Nobody really knew what to say, but at least it stopped people asking us about babies and stopped them staring at my tummy with expectancy. It also made people think a bit more carefully about how to break their own pregnancy news to us in a more sensitive way, which was appreciated. We actually wish we'd told people sooner to take the pressure off us.

All around us people were announcing their pregnancies on Facebook, by text message and sometimes, totally catching us off guard, it was done face to face. The face to face news was the hardest to cope with. I couldn't have a moment to cry or swear about how unfair things were and had to mutter out my congratulations in the most believable way I could, and then excuse myself. Don't get me wrong, I was happy for them, of course I was … my tears were just mourning the fact that I wasn't having a baby too.

Lianne Baker, UK

I went for my sperm analysis

Could not get a boner.

This actually happened to me. So not many of you will know, but the room you have to do your sperm analysis in is horrible. Well it was for me! A bin with overflowing spunk tissues and porn mags that some guy had jacked off to, all over the desk and floor. As I looked around and tried to get things started, I ran into the small (excuse the pun), problem of not getting a woody.
Lads if this happens, have no shame. Your buddy here had a non-runner too. Walk out head held high (not that head, the one on your neck), and tell reception you're doing it at home or book a hotel locally and make a day of it!

@the.swim.team

Living with infertility

It was hard every day, living with infertility
Never knowing if we'll ever have our baby
Forever the Godmother, never the Mother
Even when pregnant (at last!), constantly worried
Remembering the miscarriage we had
Thankfully, finally, after nine amazing months
Into our life came our beautiful, rainbow daughter
Let me tell others it's normal to hate this disease
It's unfair, makes you angry, frustrated and sad
Turns your life upside down, but
You carry on with your journey, living in hope.

Sheila @fertilitybooks

I'd been lost in my story

My infertility story, once private and personal, I'm now proud and thankful for. I'd felt something wasn't right. Investigations followed. Unpleasant moments. My husband and I needed ICSI (Intracytoplasmic Sperm Injection).

We embarked on what was to be a number of treatment cycles. We were fortunate to have supportive parents and trusted friends and on our first cycle, we were hopeful, yet nervous. The delivery of lots of meds, injections, hormones, waiting and the unknowns. Our first cycle failed, and there were no frozen embryos.

I carried on at work. Heavy days with personal medical appointments squeezed in. In the evening I was reading about protocols, medications, and doing a lot of over-thinking; silently absorbing others experiences via support forums online.

Socially, physically, financially, emotionally the impact was huge. Birth announcements, baby showers and gift buying, always for others. Unhelpful questioning and comments angered me. Pregnancy scan images triggered me. Bump showing, baby discussions led to tear flooded drives home. I felt angry with my body, and the immense tiredness, despair and feeling overwhelmed. Trying to think happy thoughts whilst injecting for what felt like the millionth time.

Then we experienced the sudden death of our much-loved pet. Anger and sadness flooded out. We held our lifeless pet, my husband digging a deep space in the ground, we spoke words together, which allowed us to express our previously unacknowledged grief as our sadness was beginning to be released.

Soon after, I developed cellulitis and was signed off work. My body ordered me to stop. I finally gave myself permission to rest and take stock. I'd been lost in my story.

Putting my own needs as priority was a catalyst for change and healing. I acknowledged my worth, bravery and my body, and its strength. I trusted my intuition. Around this time, I was told the magical words: 'When you start living fully the gift will come'. I was living in the present, out in the garden, enjoying holidays, friendships, spending without worry, nurturing my body and mind through Pilates, yoga and meditation. Letting go of all that was no longer serving me, allowing life and happiness in.

I began embracing situations previously so painful. Giving my mind and body the important message 'It's safe to become pregnant, surround yourself with what you wish for'.

Our next procedure, a frozen embryo transfer from a cycle the previous year felt serene. We felt calm with joyful hope, feeling accepting of the result. When our positive arrived, I didn't need a test, because I felt attuned to my body. I felt elated, but at the same time at peace.

We didn't announce our pregnancy socially until after twenty weeks. Sadly, we lost one of our twin babies along the way. We held hope that our remaining baby would flourish and grow. Our son is now three years old and helps remind us of the importance of living fully.

Claire Caldow Facebook: hopeandgrowth

From the 'Think! What Not To Say' campaign videos

"Are you sure you even want kids, because I haven't slept for five years!"

Dismissive and painful to hear – people going through a fertility journey don't care about this side of it, they are desperate to know what this tiredness feels like and to be part of the club.

#humourandcompassion

Alice Rose @thisisalicerose

From the blog: The only way out is through!

Trying to get pregnant is supposed to be a wonderful and exciting time, but for those dealing with infertility, it's a rollercoaster of emotions filled with uncertainty, grief and many feelings of loss. Infertility is stressful emotionally and physically exhausting, wearing down both the mind, body and soul. What was once so romantic and exciting quickly turns into a part-time job.

I know these feelings, because I've been there. Month after month, I experienced the loss of many failed cycles. I added all the months up, roughly eighteen of them. For eighteen months, my life stood still. It felt as if everyone around me was on the same team and I was merely a spectator watching. I felt defective and defeated. I put off doing certain things 'in case I got pregnant'. My calendar and cycle became the focus of my life and everything revolved around the fertility treatment.

Today, nine years later, I now work with individuals going through infertility. I always knew that if I made it through the journey, I would dedicate my life to help others get through it as well. It's not easy, but I found the only way out is through perseverance and a plan.

I would like to share some tools that can help support YOU in getting you through this journey.

Reduce your time on Google and social media

Most individuals struggling with a physical issue have a tendency to Google their symptoms and look for a diagnosis with the hope of understanding what is happening with their bodies. Fair enough. The problem is, three hours later, and you're still googling.

This is a maladaptive coping technique that may initially make you feel like you're taking charge of your own fertility, but often a line gets crossed, and the 'taking charge' turns into a rabbit hole. A dark one. This is the hole that sparks relentless worrying and obsessive thinking.

Social media can also have a negative effect on your well-being, making the grass look greener on the other side. It triggers your own grief to see everyone else moving on with their lives with new homes, babies, trips, engagements and good things. It's important to remember that most people only put positive experiences on social media (the things they want people to see), so it's really not an accurate depiction of what's actually happening in their lives. Consider taking a break from social media and taking control of where your attention goes.

Take control of what you can

As out of control as you may feel, there are certain things within your control. How you move your body, which expert you choose, which supplements to take, and what thoughts you choose to focus on, are just a few things within your control. These are the things you can hone in on every single day. Realize that the things you can't control, nobody else can control either, so don't worry. Part of the infertility experience is a balance between holding on and letting go. Look towards the areas that are in your power to change and let go of the rest.

Breathe

Breathing is a great way to manage anxious thoughts and reverse the stress response. When you feel yourself getting anxious, you can do a breathing technique to calm your mind and body, thereby bringing your heart rate back to normal. The breath is the link between the mind and body and can be used as an anchor whenever you need a rest. Our subconscious minds control our breathing. When we attune our conscious mind in sync with the breath, we bring ourselves back to the present.

The bigger picture

Although it may feel like infertility has taken over your life, it doesn't need to define you. You are you, not your infertility. The journey evokes a strong negative bias that protects our egos and slowly steals away hope. We must try extra hard to see the silver lining and the bigger picture. This isn't always easy, but remember you are not alone. One in six couples in Canada are struggling with infertility – and it's a similar figure whichever country you live in. The bigger picture is considering the idea of impermanence and the fact that this experience won't last forever. We change as we move through the journey and it's hard to tell who we will be at the end of it all.

My personal experience in dealing with infertility, together with my eight years of helping others face infertility, have convinced me that there are ways to cope and get through this. Many women have tried and succeeded in meeting their infertility challenges head on and you can too. In fact, you are already doing it!

Amira Posner @thefertilemind

Ours was a private infertility journey

My husband and I chose a very solitary and private infertility and IVF journey, but it was the right decision for us. Why? Well, several reasons.

My brother and sister-in-law were already on a waiting list at the same hospital for IVF where we had been referred. I was confident it would work for us both, although my husband wasn't so sure, and recommended we kept our treatment private 'just in case'. Our treatments were literally days apart. So, when we received their picture of a positive pregnancy test only two days after my period came, (confirming our unsuccessful cycle), I was actually relieved they didn't know about us. We were able to genuinely share their joy, even though we'd just had our own heart-breaking blow.

In addition, my mum hasn't got the best mental or physical health and I didn't feel she would cope with knowing our struggles as well as my brother's. My dad and his wife had come to the end of the road on their IUI and IVF journey too, and I knew she was struggling with it. So, it was best not telling them either.

My husband also felt his family would add pressure to our journey, all out of love and care, but there were questions he preferred to be without.

As we weren't telling family, we decided not to tell friends either. Only a couple of colleagues of mine eventually knew and that was because of the times I broke down in tears at work.

It's funny the conversations you are privy to when people have no idea you are going through IVF. People become 'experts' in fertility treatment because a friend's neighbour's sister went through it. It amused me on one occasion hearing, "You know, a typical IVF mum who is over protective, rushes him off to hospital with a runny nose". How I chuckled to myself over that one!

Working as a social worker certainly threw a few emotions into the mix too. I've always accepted that others can and do have children easily, even if they struggle to care for or even abuse them. That's just life. But the odd times, something would just trigger me, leave me feeling so deeply saddened that I felt I may never experience what they have. It was as if life wasn't sharing out 'luck' equally, for both me and those abused or neglected children.

There were times, I felt I may implode, carrying so much and sharing so little. Close friends faced fertility struggles too and I carried a great deal of guilt when they shared their struggles with us, yet we said nothing about ours. Yet, on the whole, I'm glad we kept our journey private. There was no burden of other people's emotions upon us, and I personally would have hated seeing friends or family eye-ball each other or change topics of conversations quickly so as not to upset or offend me, if they were talking about pregnancy or babies, for example.

As a Fertility Coach, I appreciate fully what people choose to share about their journey. It's not always through shame or guilt (as is often the assumption) that people hold back.

We are through the other side of our journey now with two happy and healthy children. Yet, my husband and I have a difference of opinion; I feel ready to talk about our IVF journey with family and friends — he does not. I respect and uphold his decision, but for me, I need a full release. He's happy for me to talk to clients or professionals as he sees the benefit of this, but for now this vision for me remains a work in progress.

ANON

Forum signature

Web forum, haven for specialist, peer support.

Anonymised and free.

Talk through a version of self-created acronyms.

The new order of things, naked reproductive histories,

Me then you.

That's the way it goes, convention in this club,

Not that I want to be a member.

Our assisted reproduction story, combined history of trying to conceive.

The list of attempts a new form of 21st century writing?

Me: mild endo. Immune issues (raised NK cells), APL, mmc 16 weeks & EPRC

OH: morp TTC: 6+ years

1st IVF: cancelled 2nd ICSI: BFN 3rd FET: BFN. Immune tx. (PUL & MC). 4th ICSI: chemical & BFN. Hysto
TTC naturally 3 mths. 5th IUI: BFN. 6th IVF: BFP!!

Justine Bold @justine_bold

Test results aren't always 'Fine'

My husband and I had been married for three years before we started trying for a baby. We both always wanted children and talked in depth about what they'd be called and what they'd be like. The excitement was electric. We almost wanted to wait, not just because of our careers, but so we had something to look forward to.

Circa May 2015 we thought: right, now is the time to get going! There was excitement and anticipation about whether we'd conceive that first month. We celebrated our thirtieth birthdays, secretly knowing we were trying for a baby. Had anyone guessed? I used to Google 'ways to surprise your husband that you're pregnant'.

Months went by and I started tracking my cycle, thinking every time my period was delayed – THIS WAS IT! I would work out the baby's due date with excitement. At the six-month mark of no pregnancy, I was panicking. I was inconsolable every time my period reared its ugly head. Friends and family started to guess we were trying, because the anxiety and stress became apparent in my face. By contrast, my husband was laid back about it. "Just relax," he'd say, "It's only been six months". I'm a worrier and I knew we wouldn't get far going to the NHS doctor, because you have to have been 'trying' for over a year to get support. I said to my husband "Let's have a fertility MOT". Neither of us had been tested and although everyone said, 'You'll be fine', that wasn't making me pregnant.

The day of the test arrived. I remember everything about that day, like it was yesterday. It was November 3rd, 2015, when we went to the fertility clinic. We had to go in for our checks at different points in the day due to sample testing and work schedules. Nervously, I got on the bed for an internal scan. They confirmed straight away that my uterus looked 'normal' and my egg reserve was 'in line with my age'. PHEW. So off to work I went, really happy that all was fine. I thought, worst case scenario, we have IVF, right? Lunchtime came and I knew my husband was being tested. Again thinking, why would anything be wrong? I looked at my watch and thought how weird it was that I hadn't heard from him. Eventually I did and bam, just like that, we knew there was a problem with his sperm, and our world came crashing down. My heart started racing a million miles a minute and I felt like I couldn't breathe.

During the 'fun' lead up to Christmas, I knew, Father Christmas definitely wasn't coming. After weeks of testing it became clear that my husband needed to undergo painful surgery for sperm extraction, known as Micro Tese. I needed to undergo IVF in tandem to extract my eggs, ready for fertilisation.

Eloise @fertility_help_hub

Resources

Below are the biographies and contact details for the contributors who wanted to be listed in case you would like to connect with them. You don't have to, but, if anything they have written resonates with you, I'm sure they would love to hear from you.

Alice Rose is an IVF-Mum and shares the positive side of her infertility journey. She is one half of catandalice.com who host live events focussing on the person, not the treatment. She is also a writer, speaker, podcaster of 'Fertility Life Raft', patient advocate and campaigner of the #twnts campaign. Alice explains: "The 'Think! What Not to Say' campaign aims to educate the wider world about how to support someone going through a fertility journey. By opening a dialogue – with humour and compassion – between patient, practitioners, family, friends, colleagues and anyone in patient facing roles, we can start to break down stigmas, normalise fertility conversations across the board and start to encourage better communication from all sides. The more we talk about it, the easier it will be for all of us".

If you want to connect with Alice:

Website www.thisisalicerose.com catandalice.com

Instagram @thisisalicerose

Amber Woodward struggled with infertility for a number of years (four to be exact) before welcoming her IVF baby into the world. She is the founder of The Preggers Kitchen where she blogs: a humourous and light-hearted website on battling infertility, that is full of positivity, action, food and laughter.

If you want to connect with Amber:

Website www.thepreggerskitchen.com

Instagram @thepreggerskitchen

Amelia Freeman is on her own infertility journey and blogs about IVF, how to support someone who is dealing with infertility, and shares real life story in her weekly 'Tube Talk'. She doesn't sugar-coat dealing with infertility, but tells it as it really is – being mad, feeling jealous, hurting.

If you want to connect with Amelia:

Website www.infertilityblows.com Instagram @infertilityblows

Amira Posner MSW, RSW and Clinical Social Worker, and her husband experienced secondary infertility. After several failed intra-uterine inseminations (IUI), Amira conceived her twins through IVF. It was her own personal experience with infertility that was the catalyst for healinginfertility.ca.

Fertility isn't just about medical intervention. Her journey has taught her about the power of the mind/body connection and using our body's intelligence to stimulate and nurture fertility. There's no magic to it. Through imagery, visualization, breathing exercises and mindfulness work, we can reverse the harmful effects of stress on the body.

She is a Clinical Social Worker with a private practice in Toronto, Ontario and has both a Bachelor and Master's Degree in Social Work from the University of Manitoba. She works with individuals and couples worldwide who are struggling with infertility. Amira developed and now facilitates the Mind-Body Fertility Group and Fab Fertile Mindfulness Fertility Series.

If you want to connect with Amira:

Website www.healinginfertility.ca Instagram @thefertilemind

Beaky Kearns is mum to three donor egg conceived daughters and is very open about her infertility story – early menopause, numerous IVF cycles and loss – in the hope that she can inspire and support others who need to consider donor eggs to have their family. She blogs about infertility and having donor conceived children and her hope is that by speaking openly, both IVF and donor conception within society will become much more open and an accepted way of starting a family.

If you want to connect with Becky:

Website www.definingmum.com

Instagram @definingmum

Claire Caldow was fortunate to find amazing support during her infertility journey, and this is why she trained to become a Freedom Fertility Coach to support individuals and couples in an easily accessible way to help them enjoy life fully again. She is incredibly proud to support others with their hope and growth.

If you want to connect with Claire:

Facebook hopeandgrowth

Dany Griffiths is the founder and creator of the Freedom Fertility Formula. She has been supporting couples with fertility issues since 2007, and has provided mentoring for specialists working in the area of fertility, pregnancy and birth since 2013. She believes the impact of infertility goes way beyond the struggle to get pregnant and have a longed-for baby, yet the importance of supporting mental health and emotional well-being is often overlooked. Sadly this emotional devastation also has the potential to affect the chances of those struggling from becoming pregnant to. Dany is on a mission to change this.

If you want to connect with Dany:
Website www.freedomfertilityformual.com
Email dany@freedomfertilityformula.com
Instagram @freedomfertilityformula

Dr Deborah Simmons had her own infertility journey before becoming the mother of two premature babies. She has provided specialized counseling for infertility-related trauma and pregnancy loss for more than twenty years. She works with fertility clinics, OB/GYN clinics, surrogacy agencies, and egg donor agencies around the United States. She provides psychoeducation to all who seek to be parents, whether this is by using IUIs, IVF, donor eggs, donor sperm, donor embryos, or gestational surrogacy. She offers clinical hypnosis, EMDR, cognitive behavioral therapy, couple's therapy, and energy work. She is also working in the area of fertility preservation with women who have been diagnosed with cancer and with transgender men and women who wish to be parents.

If you would like to connect with Dr Simmons:

Website www.partnersinfertility.net

Email drsimmons@partnersinfertility.net

Instagram @partners_in_fertility

Twitter @partnersinfert

Facebook partnersinfert

Eleanor Modral-Gibbons took charge of her health before she was even thinking about starting a family and had three children very quickly, but later went on to have two miscarriages. She is a Fertility Formula Coach.

If you would like to connect with Eleanor:

Facebook Fertility-Manchester

Website: www.fertilitymanchester.co.uk

Instagram fertility_manchester

Eloise, who experienced a difficult road to motherhood first-hand, decided to set up 'Fertility Help Hub', the fertility lifestyle hub and directory; 'an oasis of fertility'. Sign up to the newsletter for tips, support, guidance and inspiration. She wants to help break the stigma around infertility, so people don't have to suffer in silence and spend hours on Google, feeling overwhelmed.

If you want to connect with Eloise:

Instagram @fertility_help_hub,

Facebook fertilityhelphub

Website www.fertilityhelphub.co.uk

Helena Tubridy is a fertility therapist and coach, trained midwife, hypnotherapist and reflexologist. She helps couples boost their natural fertility, and prepare for IVF success, with a tailored lifestyle and emotional support programme.

If you want to connect with Helena:

Instagram @helenatubridy

Twitter @FertilityExpert

Facebook HelenaTubridyFertilityCoach

LinkedIn Helenatubridy

Jackie Figueras MSN-Ed, RN, CPC, is a passionate and accomplished registered nurse, educator, and fertility support coach. She received her training as a professional certified coach at the Institute for Professional Excellence in Coaching. Her unique combination of being a nurse, an educator, a coach and a patient who struggled with fertility issues, allow her to connect with her clients and provide engaging and interactive programs that set her apart from other communication specialists and fertility coaches. Struggling with fertility issues for years and having four consecutive miscarriages, including her daughters' twin, has created a deeper passion for changing healthcare and the fertility journey for many women. She truly understands the impact stress can have on your physical, mental and emotional health and is dedicated to helping guide women on their own journeys to find more balance and peace.

If you want to connect with Jackie:

Instagram @thesupportivemama,

Email jackie@thesupportivemama.com

Website www.thesupportivemama.com

Justine Bold has personal experience of infertility as she had a 12 year journey to motherhood, finally becoming a mum to twin boys in her forties. She has written articles on infertility and edited a book entitled 'Integrated approaches to infertility, IVF and recurrent miscarriage' that was published in 2016, and co-written a book on mental health that was published in 2019. She works as a University Lecturer and has research interests in lifestyle and nutrition and their links to health problems, such as endometriosis and polycystic ovarian syndrome.

If you want to connect with Justine:

Twitter @justineboldfood

Instagram justinebold

Website www.worcester.ac.uk/about/profiles/justine-bold

Karmenn Wennerlind is an infertility warrior, miscarriage survivor, mama to three rainbow miracles and one furbaby

If you want to connect with Karmenn:

Instagram @karmennwennerlind

Kate Davies RN, BSc(Hons), FP Cert, Fertility Nurse Consultant, has over twenty years experience in fertility and women's health. She has also undertaken specialist training in PCOS, and has helped hundreds of women control their symptoms and go on to conceive. She is a qualified Fertility Coach and offers her patients much needed emotional support as well as clinical advice.

If you want to connect with Kate:

Instagram @your_fertility_journey

Website www.yourfertilityjourney.com

Email Kate@yourfertilityjourney.com

Facebook YourFertilityJourney

Twitter fertjourney

Pinterest yourfertilityjourney

Lauren Manaker MS, RDN, LD, CLEC is a registered and licensed dietitian-nutritionist who resides in Charleston, South Carolina, USA. She focuses on fertility, preconception, and prenatal nutrition and has a passion for interpreting data for the general public to understand. She recently published a book for men who want to learn more about how diet and lifestyle play a role in fertility called 'Fueling Male Fertility', and is available on Amazon.com.

If you want to connect with Lauren:

Instagram @LaurenManaker_RDN

Nicola Headley supports women and couples with a unique mix of counselling, coaching and mind/body techniques to regain emotional control of their fertility journey and enhance their chances of fertility success.

If you want to connect with Nicola:

Website www.nicolaheadley.com

Instagram @nicola_freedomfertility

Facebook Nicola Headley Freedom Fertility Formula Specialist

Nicola Salmon is a fat-positive and feminist fertility coach. She advocates for change in how fat women are treated on their fertility journey. She supports fat women, and others with disordered eating, who are struggling to get pregnant, to find peace with their body, find their own version of health and finally escape the yo-yo dieting cycle. For more information download: *The Fat Girl's Guide to Getting Pregnant:*

http://nicolasalmon.co.uk/fat-girls-guide-getting-pregnant/

If you want to connect with Nicola:

Instagram @fatpositivefertility

Website www.nicolasalmon.co.uk

Rachel Cathan is the author of the book: *336 Hours* – a diary of one woman's battle through infertility and IVF during her five-year quest for motherhood. The story is set within the pressure cooker of the narrator's third, and supposedly final, IVF treatment, Rachel is also a fertility counsellor.

If you want to connect with Rachel:

Website www.Rachelcathan.co.uk

Facebook 336hours

Twitter rachelcathan

Salise Wright is the founder of Lohojo - Producers of affirmation calendars

If you want to connect with Salise:

Website www.lohojo.co.uk

Email hello@lohojo.co.uk

Facebook Lohojo.uk

Instagram Lohojo.uk

Sandi Friedlos helps women manage the emotional upheaval caused by fertility frustrations and challenges in trying to have a baby, so they are free from feeling their life is 'on hold' playing the waiting game.

If you want to connect with Sandi:

Website www.sandifriedlos.com

Email sandi@sandifriedlos.com

Instagram @sandifriedlos

Twitter sandifriedlos

Facebook SandiFriedlos

Sarah Rollandini and her husband had a long journey to have their family, which included fertility meds, a tubal pregnancy and miscarriage. Their children finally joined them through domestic adoption and gestational surrogacy. She is a blogger and writer.

If you want to connect with Sarah:

Website www.sarahrollandini,

Instagram @infertility_cheerleader

Facebook sarahrollandini

Twitter SarahRollandini

Stephanie Roth Your Fertile Self. Holistic Fertility Coach. Certified Holistic Counsellor, has completed the Optimal Fertility program with Integrative Women's Health Institute and is a Certified Holistic Health Coach. She says: "I had my own fertility rollercoaster journey before taking charge of my nutrition and lifestyle. Our next intra-uterine insemination (IUI) cycle was a success".

If you want to connect with Stephanie:

Website www.yourfertileself.com

Facebook www.facebook.com/yourfertileself

Twitter www.twitter.com/YourFertileSelf

Instagram @yourfertileself

Tori Day author of the book: *Warrior: Battling infertility –*

staying sane while trying to conceive. Tori had her own rollercoaster infertility journey; 'Warrior' is her first book as an Indie author.

If you want to connect with Tori:

Twitter @ToriDayWrite

Thank you for reading

Would you like to help others on their TTC journey? You can by leaving a review about this book on the online store you purchased it from.

How great is that?!

Sheila Lamb